The Eye and Foot in Diabetes

Edited by Jeffery Grigsby and Fethi Derbel

Published in London, United Kingdom

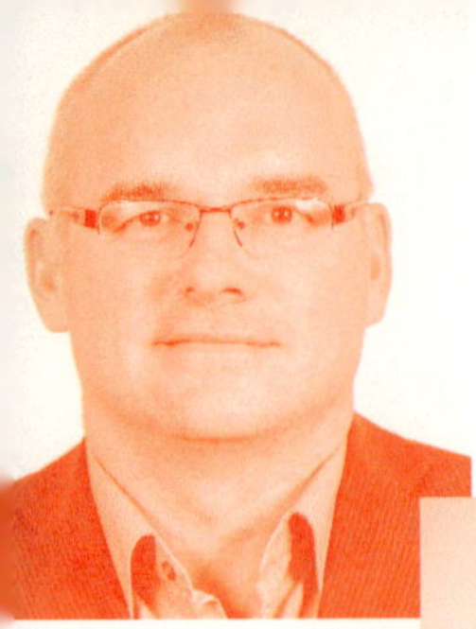
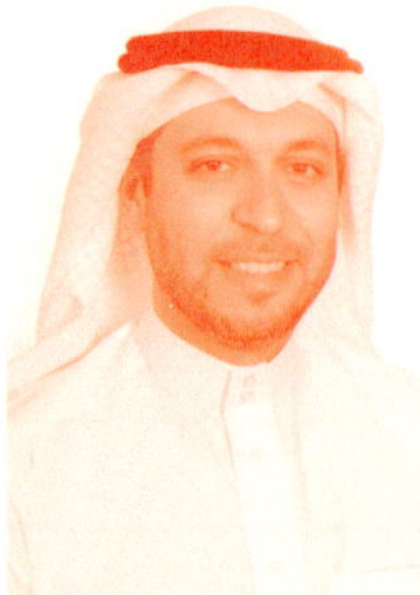
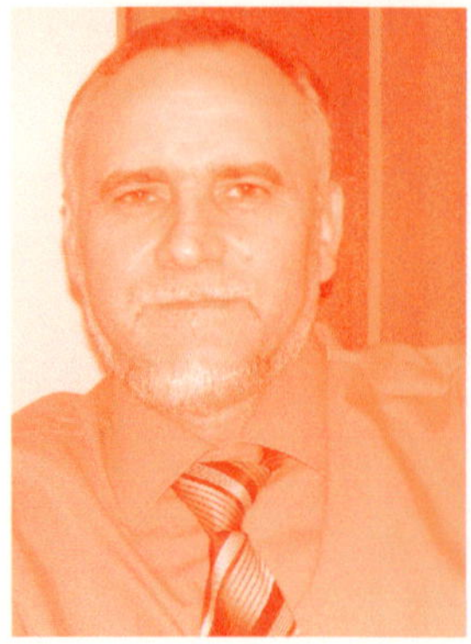
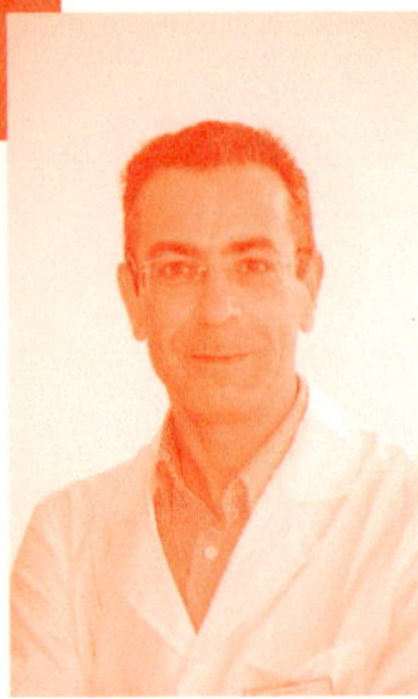
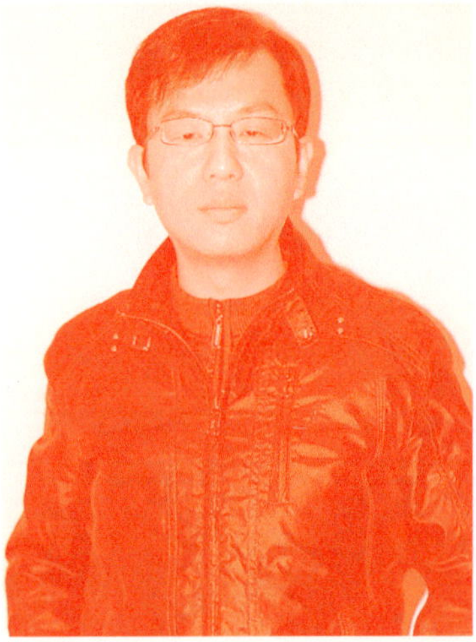
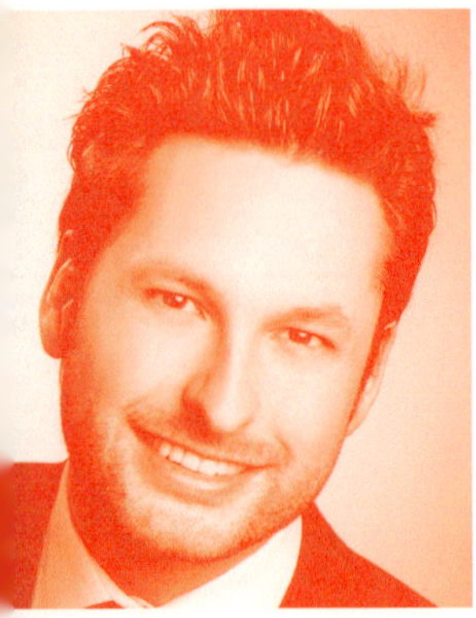
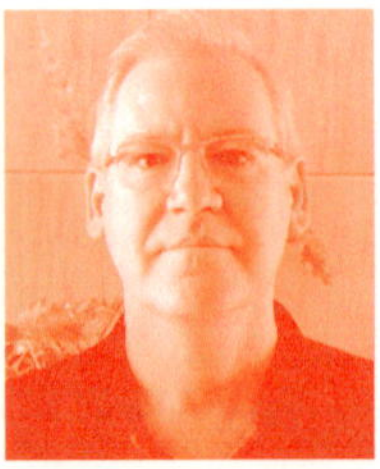

IntechOpen

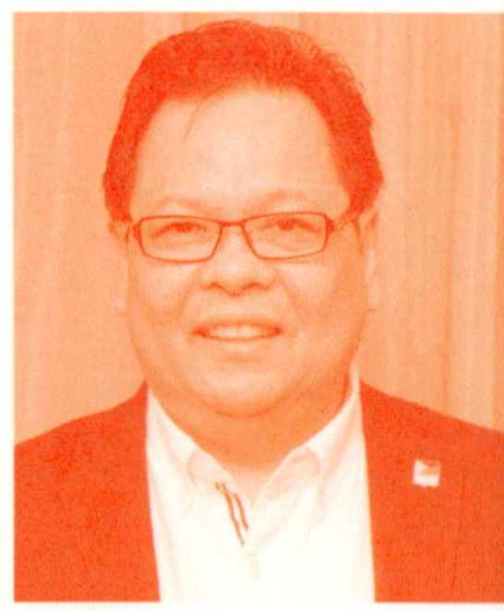
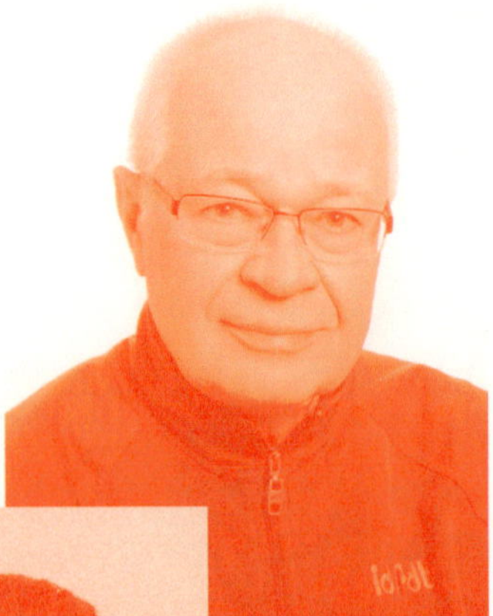
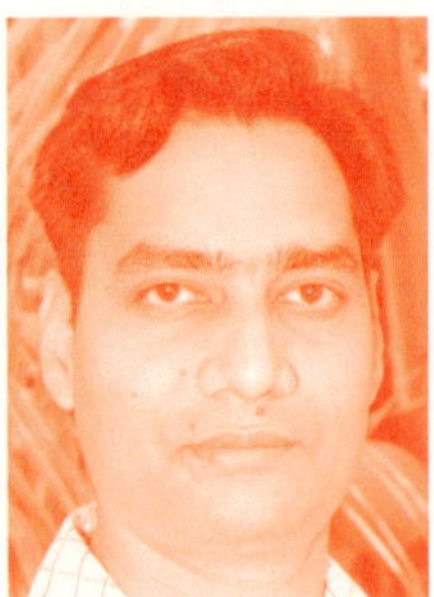
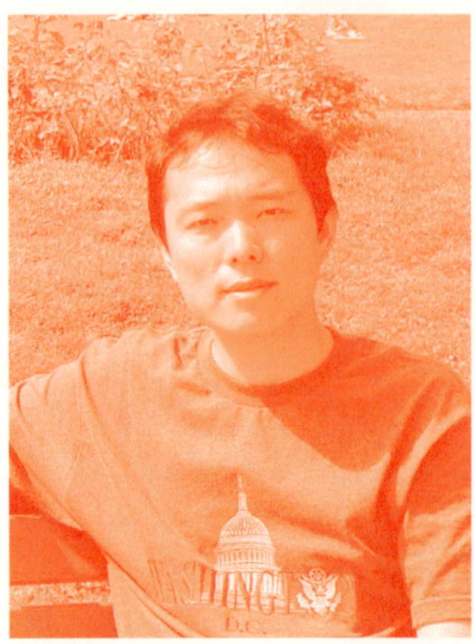
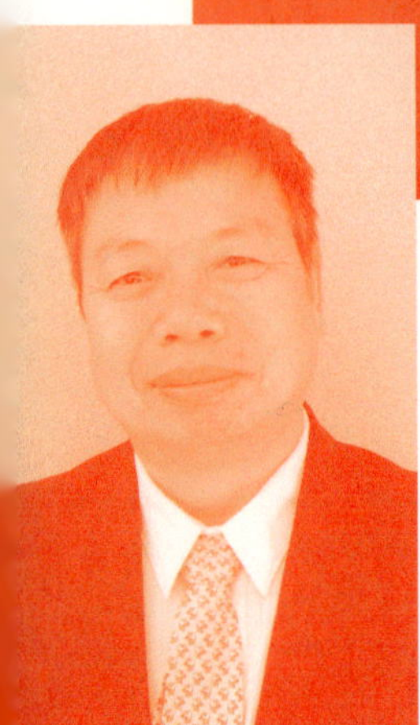
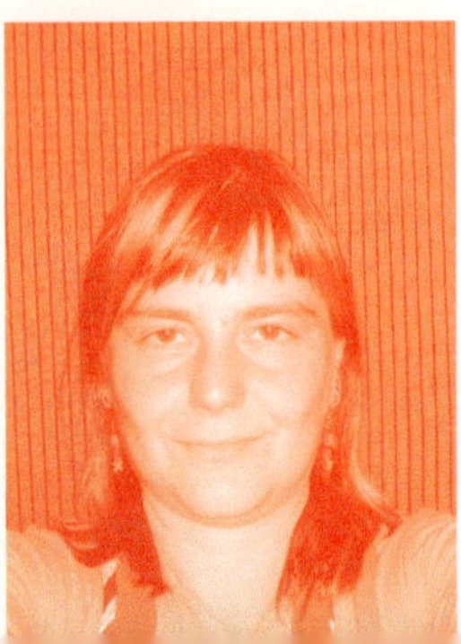

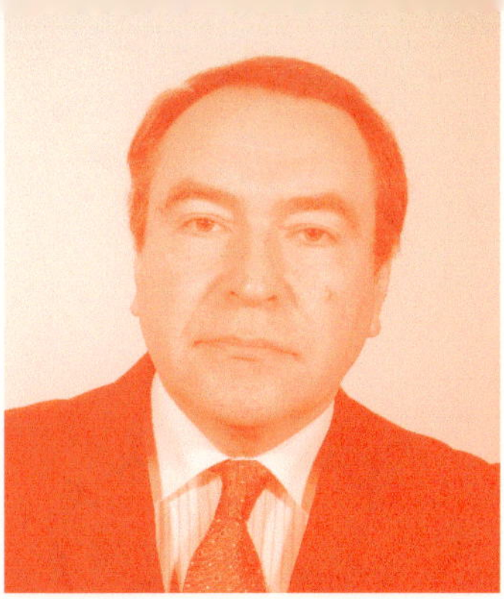
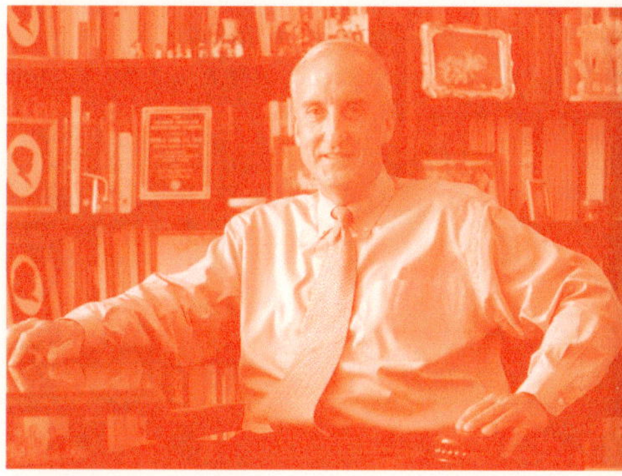
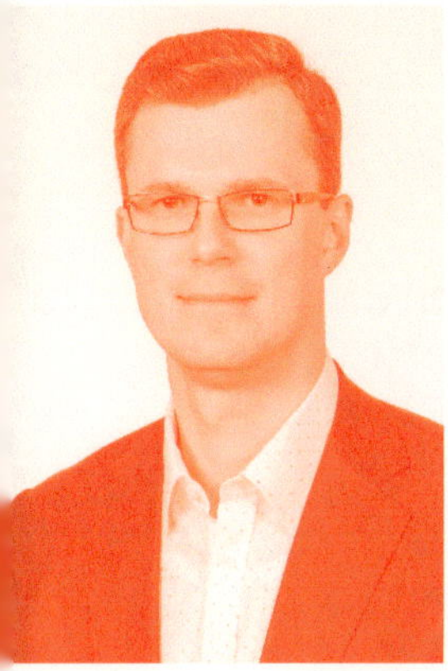
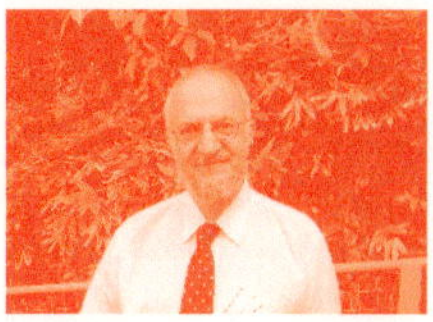
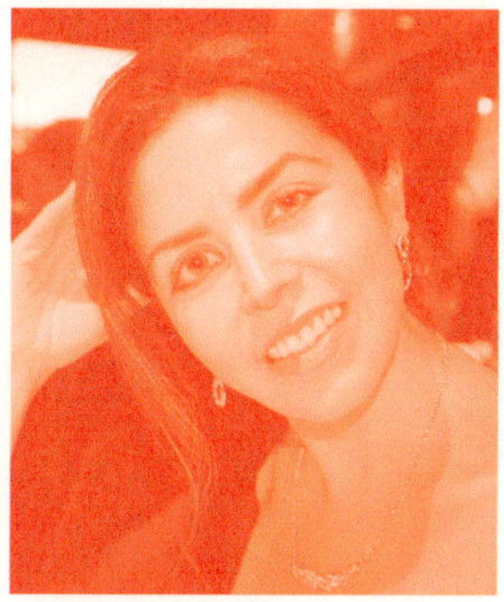

Supporting open minds since 2005

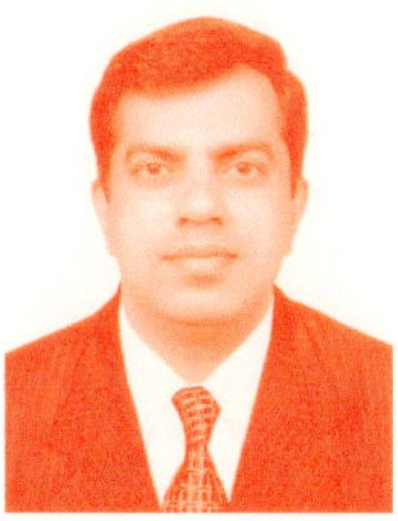
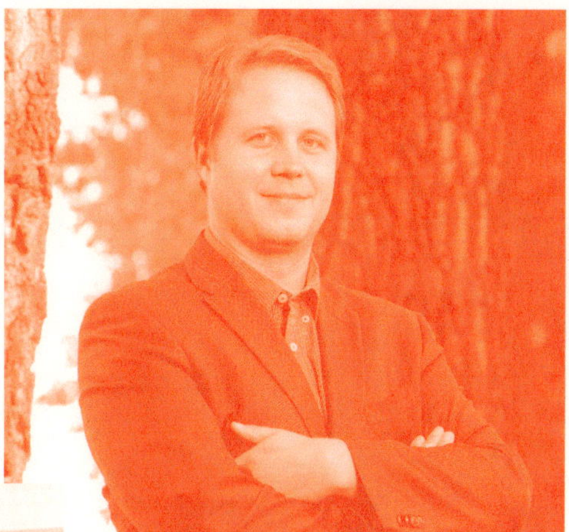
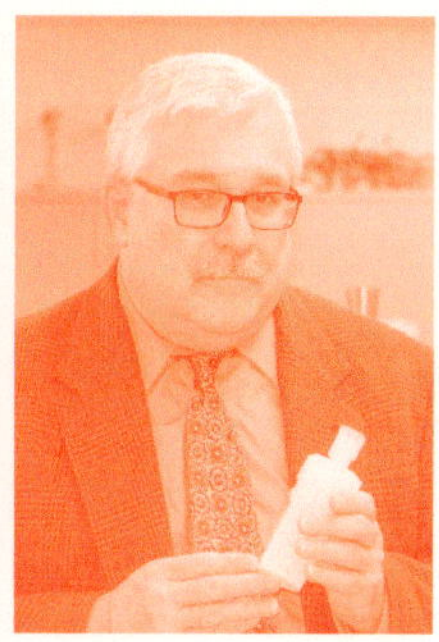
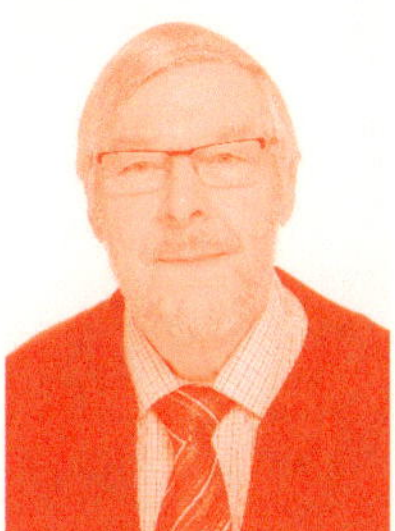
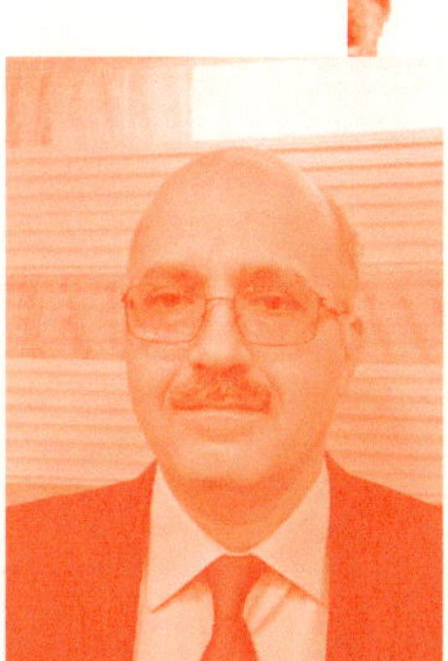
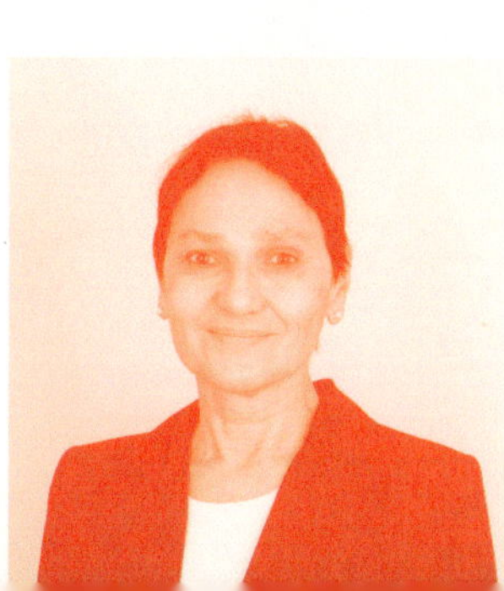
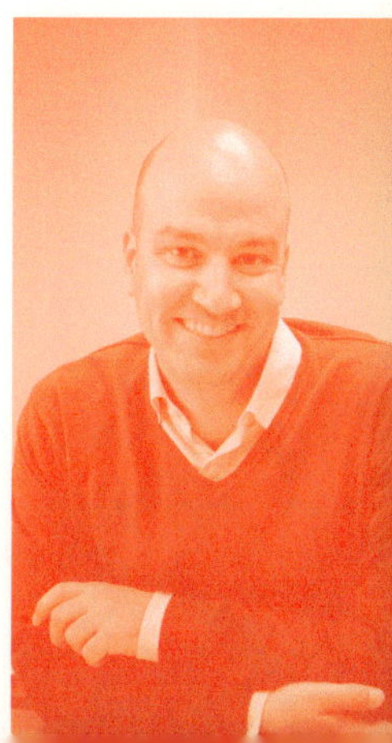

The Eye and Foot in Diabetes
http://dx.doi.org/10.5772/intechopen.83159
Edited by Jeffery Grigsby and Fethi Derbel

Contributors
Laura Valdez, XinYee Ooi, Rujman Khan, Matthew Parvus, Andrew Tsin, Jacqueline M Lopes De Faria, Marcella N Dátilo, Ogugua Okonkwo, Caroline Fisher, Maria Pilar Vela-Orus, María Sonia Gaztambide-Sáenz, Suresh K.S., Sukesh Kumar A., Atamjit Singh, Kirandeep Kaur, Shivani Attri, Danish Malhotra, Aditi Verma, Neena Bedi, Preet Mohinder Singh Bedi, Fanna Liu, Chung-Lun Lu, Shiu-Nan Chen, Yu-Sheng Wu, Ya-Chih Chang, Sherwin Chen, Imran Ali Shaikh, Naila Siddiqui, Javeria Shaikh, Fethi Derbel, Meriem Braiki, Mohamed Ali Khalifa, Bilel Faidi, Mosaab Ghannouchi, Lianghong Yin

First published in London, United Kingdom, 2020 by IntechOpen
IntechOpen is the global imprint of INTECHOPEN LIMITED, registered in England and Wales, registration number: 11086078, 5 Princes Gate Court, London, SW7 2QJ, United Kingdom
Printed in Croatia

British Library Cataloguing-in-Publication Data
A catalogue record for this book is available from the British Library

Additional hard and PDF copies can be obtained from orders@intechopen.com

The Eye and Foot in Diabetes
Edited by Jeffery Grigsby and Fethi Derbel
p. cm.
Print ISBN 978-1-83880-944-7
Online ISBN 978-1-83880-945-4
eBook (PDF) ISBN 978-1-83880-946-1

For EU product safety concerns:
IN TECH d.o.o., Prolaz Marije Krucifikse Kozulić 3, 51000 Rijeka, Croatia, info@intechopen.com or visit our website at intechopen.com.

Meet the editors

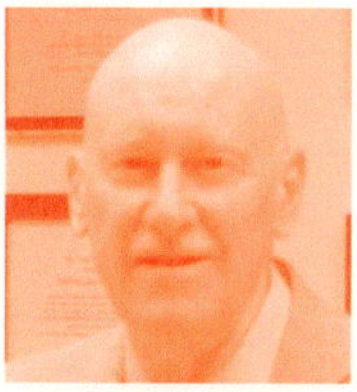

Dr. Jeff Grigsby practiced in ophthalmology and optometry practices in West Texas several years before founding Vision Health Specialties. He saw patients, lectured on eye disease, and dabbled in eye care politics. A mid-career change sent him back to school in biology with an emphasis in diabetic retinal disease. Since that time working as an optometrist, teacher, and biologist, he continues to see patients and manage a large eye care practice. Additionally, he works as a clinic director of a laser refractive center, lectures on diabetic retinopathy and refractive surgical issues, performs clinical and basic science research, writes research and literature reviews on the biological roots of diabetic eye disease, and edits papers and books on diabetic retinopathy.

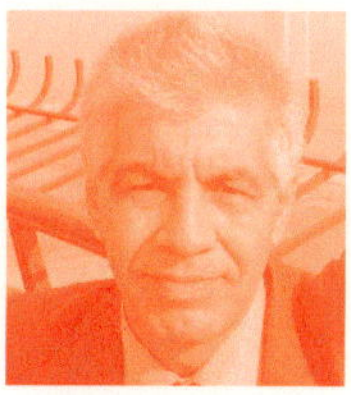

Professor Fethi Derbel was born in 1960 in Tunisia. He received his medical degree from the Sousse Faculty of Medicine at Sousse, University of Sousse, Tunisia. He completed his surgical residency in General Surgery at the University Hospital Farhat Hached of Sousse and was a member of the Unit of Liver Transplantation in the University of Rennes, France. He then worked in the Department of Surgery at the Sahloul University Hospital in Sousse. Professor Derbel is presently working at the Clinique les Oliviers, Sousse, Tunisia. His hospital activities are mostly concerned with laparoscopic, colorectal, pancreatic, hepatobiliary, and gastric surgery. He is also very interested in hernia surgery and performs ventral hernia repairs and inguinal hernia repairs. He has been a member of the GREPA and Tunisian Hernia Society (THS). During his residency, he managed patients suffering from diabetic foot, and he was very interested in this pathology. For this reason, he decided to coordinate a book project dealing with the diabetic foot. Professor Derbel has published many articles in journals and collaborates intensively with IntechOpen Access Publisher as an editor.

Contents

Preface

Much work has been done in an attempt to understand the mechanisms of disease in the eyes and feet of those who live with diabetes. On July 27, 1921, Banting and Best recovered insulin from a dog pancreas. Previously those diagnosed with type 1 diabetes gradually withered away and died within a year. It was thought that finally a cure was found for what we now refer to as type 1 diabetes. Now we struggle with what was unforeseen at the time, the long-term effects of hyperglycemia in those who have either type 1 or type 2 diabetes. Diabetic retinopathy remains the leading cause of blindness in working age adults around the world. In addition, the foot issues and potential amputation of those who struggle with diabetes are well known and remain a struggle for both patients and providers.

This book covers a range of issues on both the eyes and feet of those with diabetes. The eye section of the book details the molecular and biological origins of diabetic eye disease as well as a chapter on vitrectomy for diabetic retinopathy. The section on the foot also outlines mechanisms of disease, evaluation methods of the diabetic foot, and its association with kidney and neurologic disease.

We are grateful to those contributors who have worked to make this book a reality. It has been an honor to present the work of such a distinguished group of scientists, clinicians, and surgeons. The staff at IntechOpen has also patiently contributed to actualizing this project. It is our hope that these efforts will enable a further understanding of the mechanisms by which diabetes affects not only the eyes and feet, but how that relates to other parts of the body.

Jeff Grigsby
Vision Health Specialties,
Texas Tech University Health Science Center,
University of Houston, College of Optometry,
Texas, USA

Fethi Derbel
Clinique les Oliviers,
Tunisia

Section 1

The Eye in Diabetes

Chapter 1

Advanced Glycation End Products: Formation, Role in Diabetic Complications, and Potential in Clinical Applications

Rujman Khan, Xin Yee Ooi, Matthew Parvus, Laura Valdez and Andrew Tsin

Abstract

Hyperglycemic conditions and disruptions to glucose-regulating pathways lead to increased formation of highly reactive aldehydes, methylglyoxal and glyoxal, which react with certain arginine and lysine residues in proteins to form advanced glycation end products (AGEs). These AGEs damage the integrity of the retinal vasculature predominantly through two mechanisms: non-receptor-mediated damage, which pertains to the interaction with extracellular matrix and its functional properties, and receptor-mediated damage through AGE interactions with their receptors (RAGE) on pericytes and Muller cells. Damage occurring between AGE and RAGE potentially generates reactive oxygen species, inflammatory cytokines, and growth factors. Both mechanisms result in increased permeability of endothelial tight junctions, and this increased permeability can lead to leaking and eventually ischemia. Once this ischemia becomes significant, neovascularization can occur, the hallmark of proliferative diabetic retinopathy. Current pharmaceutical studies have shown the potential of AGE inhibitors, such as aminoguanidine, in decreasing AGE production, thus minimizing its effects in hyperglycemic conditions. Other pharmaceutical interventions, such as Tanshinone IIA, aim to protect cells from the impacts of AGEs. Future research will not only continue to understand the properties of AGEs and their effects on diabetes and diabetic complications like diabetic retinopathy but will also explore how they impact other diseases.

Keywords: advanced glycation end products, oxoaldehyde, RAGE, hyperglycemia, diabetic retinopathy, inflammation, cytokine, neovascularization

1. Introduction

Advanced glycation end products (AGEs) are formed through a non-enzymatic process in hyperglycemic conditions, and they impact the retinal vasculature negatively through the formation of reactive oxygen species, secretion of aberrant proteins or growth factors, alteration of the extracellular matrix, and secretion of inflammatory cytokines [1]. It is important to consider the difficulty of differentiating the effects of hyperglycemia from those of AGEs, as AGE concentration is controlled by glucose levels. Because of this, occasionally high glucose levels are measured interchangeably with high levels of AGEs. There are two primary mechanisms by which AGEs damage the retinal vasculature which will be discussed in this chapter: interactions with RAGE (AGE receptors) and damage to the extracellular matrix [2]. While these two mechanisms work differently, both pathways result in thickening of the basement membrane which impairs signaling between cells of the microvasculature hindering their structure and increasing rigidity, which leads to the hemorrhagic signs seen in patients with diabetic retinopathy (DR) [3]. Endogenous anti-stressors are important for the management of high levels of AGEs through various mechanisms, but many times are not sufficient to control the progression of DR [2]. Thus, it is important to modify the production of AGEs through exogenous mechanisms, such as nutrition, reducing smoking, or treating the condition through medication [2].

2. AGE formation

Advanced glycation end products (AGEs) were first discovered in the early 1900s by the Maillard reaction process. Scientists discovered that when amino acids were heated in a mixture with reducing sugars, the reaction turned a yellowish brown color. Further studies indicated that reducing sugars, i.e., glucose, reacted non-enzymatically with the amino acid reagents to form Schiff bases, an early glycation product, and Amadori products, intermediate glycation products. AGE formation can utilize other reagents such as lipids, connective tissue extracellular matrix, and nucleic acids. The process of glycation is enhanced by diabetic complications and occurs in the earlier stages of the Maillard reaction; intracellular sugars, such as glycolytic pathway intermediate glucose-6-phosphate, are glycated at a faster rate than glucose. Amadori products are α-dicarbonyls (oxoaldehydes) such as 3-deoxyglucosone (3-DG) and methylglyoxal (MGO) which is formed by the non-oxidative rearrangement of Amadori adducts from fructose-3-phosphate in the polyol pathway. This pathway has also been studied as a precursor to hyperglycemia-induced damage in diabetes. Methylglyoxal and 3-deoxyglucosone are formed in the early stages of glycation processes: degradation of glucose, Schiff's bases, and from Amadori products; these oxoaldehyde products can serve as a checkpoint in the AGE pathway since an accumulation of these products is an implication of accelerated vascular damage [4, 5].

3. Mechanism of action

The main mechanisms of AGE that affect cells are the adducts on proteins (including N-carboxymethyllysine, pentosidine, or hydroimidazolone) that can interact via AGE ligand-gated receptors such as RAGE on endothelium that lead to secretion of cytokines TNF-α and VEGF; AGEs can stem from exogenous and endogenous adducts due to glucose metabolism. RAGE is the most widely studied AGE receptor found on endothelial cells in vasculature and on macrophages and microglia. AGE interacts with RAGE on macrophages, leading to intracellular generation of free radicals and oxidative stress, which are then phosphorylated by MAP kinase to activate NF-κB and increase expression of NF-κB controlled genes to cause vasoconstriction, enhanced adhesion molecule expression, and induce a procoagulant state. An overexpression of RAGE leads to oxidative stress and NF-κB activation. Current studies show that cross-linked AGEs with RAGE on proteins are closely linked with diabetic retinopathy progression. In the diabetic retina, AGE and adducts are found on vascular cells, neurons, glia, and in elevated levels in Muller macroglia—these specialized retinal cells show increased dysfunction in hyperglycemic and hypoxic conditions that lead to more AGE formation. AGEs induce oxidative stress and consequent apoptosis of retinal pericytes; furthermore, AGEs induce the closure of intercellular junctions between endothelial cells [4–7].

3.1 AGE-RAGE interactions

Inflammation is an important component in the progression of diabetic retinopathy (DR), and AGEs induce this process through interaction with receptors on the cell surface called RAGEs. These receptors are found on most cells, meaning that AGEs exert a wide effect on many different organs. In DR, results of AGE-RAGE interaction on inflammatory cells such as macrophages and lymphocytes, and on microvascular cells such as endothelial cells or pericytes are thought to produce a significant impact on the progression of DR [8]. Monocytes and lymphocytes secrete inflammatory cytokines through the induction of NF-κB [9], production of IL-1, IL-6, IL-8, MCP-1 and TNF-α, and upregulation of adhesion molecules such as VCAM and ICAM [9]. IL-8 and TNF-α levels are elevated in patients with nonproliferative diabetic retinopathy (NPDR), signifying the increased inflammation in the early stages of DR. These cytokines are produced by activated neuronal cells and endothelial cells, and they exert their effect by causing early neuronal cell death in the retina [9]. Inflammation negatively impacts the retinal vasculature by altering the action of vascular cells which leads to the upregulation of various proteins that contribute to the thickening of the basement membrane. MIP-1, IL-3, and IL-1 are thought to play a role in angiogenesis [9, 10], which would facilitate the progression from NPDR to proliferative diabetic retinopathy (PDR). Communication between glial cells and neurons is imperative for maintenance of the vasculature, and it has been shown that inflammation can impede the crosstalk between these cells early in the disease process [9]. Thickening of the basement membrane is one of the leading mechanisms by which crosstalk amongst cells of the retinal vasculature are impeded. This crosstalk is essential for many processes such as providing energy to retinal vascular cells and maintaining homeostasis [9]. In endothelial cells, AGE-RAGE interaction has been shown to increase proliferation via increased VEGF production induced through the MAPK pathway [10, 11]. This process contributes to angiogenesis and accelerates the progression of DR from NPDR to PDR. In pericytes, an opposite effect has been observed, as increased AGE-RAGE interaction leads to apoptosis of these cells, which is one of the first steps in the pathogenesis of DR [11]. As pericyte dropout occurs, the vasculature becomes less regulated leading to hemorrhage and leaking.

3.2 Oxidative stress

Reactive oxygen species (ROS) accumulate in DR from the conversion of glucose to fructose through the NADPH pathway. This accumulation of ROS leads to increased production of AGEs, which then exert their effects through AGE-RAGE interactions or by crosslinking extracellular matrix proteins. One of the outcomes of AGE-RAGE interactions is production of ROS as well, leading to enhanced concentrations of ROS and further progression of the disease. Aldose reductase, which is upregulated to compensate for the high levels of glucose and is essential for the conversion of glucose to fructose, activates a serine/threonine-related protein kinase PKC-δ. Protein kinase PKC-δ is known to inhibit platelet derived growth factor survival activity, an essential pathway for pericyte proliferation and survival. Considering that pericyte loss is typically the initial step in the pathogenesis of DR, this explains the role of ROS in the early stages of DR [12].

3.3 Impact on the extracellular matrix

The other predominant mechanism of damage from AGEs pertains to their effect on the extracellular matrix of the retinal basement membrane. Inflammation induced by AGEs that was discussed above has a significant impact on the basement membrane, specifically from the elevated levels of inflammatory cytokines IL-1β and TNF-α which induce the production of extracellular matrix proteins. As these excess proteins accumulate in the extracellular matrix, the basement membrane begins to thicken. When AGEs attach to collagen or elastin in the extracellular matrix, it causes the collagen to be less susceptible to hydrolytic breakdown and becomes less flexible. It has also been found that glycation increases the production of collagen and other extracellular matrix proteins, along with the increase in production induced by inflammatory cytokines. This increased production and crosslinking of collagen along with the decreased elastin levels significantly increase the rigidity of the microvasculature through stiffening and thickening of the basement membrane [2, 10, 13].

The accumulation and crosslinking of extracellular matrix proteins contributes to the thickening of the basement membrane, which hinders its integrity ultimately leading to the hemorrhagic pathologies that occur as a result of diabetic retinopathy. The initial damage caused by this thickening is decreased perfusion of the retinal capillaries, leading to occlusion or degeneration of these capillaries [14]. This is one of the characteristic steps in NPDR: ischemia caused by lack of oxygen perfusion sets off the cascade of events that leads to neovascularization, the hallmark of PDR. When looking at the sequelae following the impact of AGEs on the basement membrane, it suggests that AGEs play a significant role in the progression and pathogenesis of diabetic retinopathy. A study showed rats with diabetes tested positive for AGEs (periodic acid/Schiff reagent positive material) at significantly higher levels than those under normal conditions [15]. Rats with diabetes also demonstrated a twofold increase in acellular retinal capillaries over the course of 26 weeks compared to their wild type counterparts, and diabetic rats also experienced significant capillary closure over the course of 75 weeks.

4. Dietary and exogenous sources

Processing of foods at high temperatures using the Maillard reaction to enhance flavoring and color subsequently leads to the formation of reactive aldehydes that leads to formation of advanced glycation end products, which are also formed naturally in body tissues. Studies depicted that canned meats, nuts, and grain-based products contained the highest levels of AGE, and coffee, butter, vegetables, and fruits as well as food prepared by steaming or boiling contained the lowest amounts of AGE [5, 16].

Research studies show that the average amount of AGE consumed on a daily basis by an individual range from 12,000 to 20,000 kilo-units (kU) of AGEs/day with diabetic subjects consuming a range of 4000–24,000 kU AGEs/day. Pyrraline is one of the most common AGE adducts and may be found in milk and bread crust, while pentosidine, another AGE adduct, is found in pretzel sticks and in its free form in coffee. Study of individual AGEs suggest that protein-bound pentosidine is not as readily absorbed as free pentosidine, therefore, increased levels free AGE in urine and plasma is correlated to AGE-rich dietary intake. Intake of elevated levels of sodium, carbohydrates, and vitamins were found to not be associated with DR risk or progression. Relationship between dietary AGE and promotion of AGE formation in the body tissues will require new research since current research has only centered on skin autofluorescence before and after intake of AGE-rich foods [5, 16].

The effects of dietary AGE were examined in several studies. AGE-poor diets depicted improved biomarkers for oxidative stress, endothelial, and inflammation in healthy subjects, and restricted AGE diets showed decreased levels of oxidative stress in diabetic patients as well as decreased insulin resistance and reduced levels of low-density-lipoprotein. Other studies have also found that dietary AGEs affect inflammatory markers including cytokine TNF-α, and AGE-poor diets have led to decreased risk for cardiovascular disease and endothelial dysfunction. Several studies have also examined the effects of dietary AGE on motor functions, finding that increases in oxidative stress and inflammation due to high levels of AGE lead to muscle stiffness and loss of elasticity [5, 16].

5. Physiological alterations due to hyperglycemic conditions

Hyperglycemic conditions initiate formation of AGE and promote biochemical abnormalities that involve formation of AGE. The three main AGE formation biochemical abnormalities include flux via hexosamine pathway, diacylglycerol-mediated activation of PKC-β with benfotiamine, and the stimulation of transketolase activity that induces excess triose phosphates to undergo the pentose phosphate pathway [17, 18].

The primary precursor of AGE is glucose, but other carbonyl precursors exists, though diminutively less reactive, including glyoxal, methylglyoxal, and 3-deoxyglucosone that result from glycolysis. The levels of AGE in the body tissues increase significantly in complications of disease such as diabetic retinopathy, but it is the accumulation of AGE that results in accelerated complications of diseases. Body cells have innate detoxification systems that prevent accumulation of AGE precursors such as methylglyoxal, and detoxification properties of enzymes may be essential in further research about prevention of diabetic retinopathy complications. Deterioration of kidney function leads to accumulation of AGEs, thus leading to endothelial abnormality and vascular disease [4, 5, 17].

6. Treatments

No cure for diabetic retinopathy has been discovered yet, despite many efforts from various clinical trials. The standard pharmacological treatment currently for diabetic retinopathy is anti-VEGF injections, which aids in the stabilization and halts progression of the disease [19]. This approach has only been successful in treating about two-thirds of the population and the best second-line pharmacological therapy has not been identified [19]. These factors have spurred the search for a better alternative, especially agents which combat the AGEs and their effects directly. There are different categories of treatments against AGEs, but the most widely studied treatments include those that specifically inhibit AGEs themselves as well as lifestyle changes to reduce the production of AGEs.

6.1 Direct AGE inhibitors

The first direct AGE inhibitor that garners the most promise is aminoguanidine, which inhibits AGE formation on both collagen and the basement membrane [15]. As discussed above in the section about AGE's impact on the extracellular matrix, AGEs crosslink collagen and other proteins in the basement membrane and extracellular matrix which causes it to thicken, lose its integrity and ultimately become leaky. By inhibiting the formation of these crosslinked proteins, the basement membrane and extracellular matrix can preserve their integrity and the normal communication between pericytes and endothelial cells can continue. A study demonstrated that rats treated with aminoguanidine showed significantly less AGE deposition in the basement membrane/extracellular matrix and overall healthier capillaries [15]. Treatment with aminoguanidine also reduced endothelial cell proliferation in diabetic retina, which is another pathological change associated with diabetes. The downside is that this treatment was unable to completely resolve all of the pathological processes of diabetes, namely the occurrence of retinal microaneurysms. In untreated diabetic rats, 38% demonstrated microaneurysms while those treated with aminoguanidine reduced the incidence to 20% (0% in controls). This improvement is promising, but microaneurysms lead to vessel destruction, which advances the progression of NPDR to PDR, the more detrimental stage of DR. An alternative study demonstrated an even greater decrease in microaneurysms, but their sample size was small (a single retina) and it was conducted in dogs rather than rats [20].

Another direct AGE inhibitor is pyridoxamine. This compound has been found to decrease glycation of proteins in the extracellular matrix as well as decrease the formation and production of AGEs. A study measured the success of treating diabetic retinopathy with pyridoxamine by the quantity of acellular capillaries formed over a period of time [4]. Acellular capillaries are nonperfused capillaries which result from a variety of factors onset by diabetes such as pericyte dropout, extracellular matrix, and endothelial damage [21]. After 29 weeks, it was found that diabetic rats treated with pyridoxamine showed similar amounts of acellular capillaries to controls. It also demonstrated the impact of pyridoxamine on the production of extracellular matrix proteins, which are upregulated in diabetic retinopathy. Pyridoxamine significantly reduced the production of extracellular matrix proteins like collagen type IV and laminin, close to the levels found in controls [4].

6.2 Other pharmaceutical interventions

Besides the usage of direct AGE inhibitors, other drugs options are being explored. One such drug is Tanshinone IIA (Tan IIA). Tan IIA is derived from the roots of *Salvia miltiorrhiza*, which is a plant that is used in traditional Chinese medicine. Studies indicate that Tan IIA impacts several of the negative effects that hyperglycemic conditions have on human retinal endothelial cells. Tan IIA has an inhibitory effect on proliferation, migration, and vascularization in human endothelial cells and has some correlation to VEGF expression [22]. In terms of AGEs, a recent study explored how Tan IIA protects retinal endothelial cells from the impacts of AGEs, specifically cell dysfunction resulting from the presence of MGO. The study showed that MGO impacted cell viability negatively in a dose-dependent manner. Treatment of the cells with Tan IIA increased their viability in conditions where MGO was also present. MGO presence also resulted in mitochondrial fission in bovine retinal endothelial cells, and the presence of Tan IIA protected against this type of AGE-induced injury in the cells [23].

6.3 Lifestyle modification

Exogenous AGEs are AGEs that are consumed and produced through diet and lifestyle, and they differ from the endogenous AGEs that form in hyperglycemic conditions metabolically. Because of this, diet and lifestyle changes are arguably the most important treatment in DR, as diet is a significant contributor to exogenous AGEs found in the form of foods high in protein and fat. Pertaining to lifestyle, smoking tobacco products is associated with higher levels of AGEs in serum which contributes to the progression and risk of DR [24]. Overall, a decreased calorie intake, a modified diet, and smoking cessation have been shown to increase risk and overall disease progression of DR and should be an important treatment regimen, in addition to pharmacological treatments with AGE inhibitors, in all patients with DR.

7. Conclusion

Advanced glycation end products (AGEs) are formed in increasing amounts due to hyperglycemic conditions implicated in diseases such as diabetic retinopathy. Endogenous AGEs are products from metabolic pathways that follow the Maillard reaction with the oxidation of oxoaldehydes. Exogenous AGEs may come from food sources processed at high temperatures, which increased the amount of reactive aldehydes in the food. Several studies have indicated that inhibition of AGEs holds high potential in the treatment of diabetic retinopathy. Aminoguanidine, a nonspecific inhibitor of AGE, holds the most pharmaceutical promise according to several studies conducted, but other drugs such as Tanshinone IIA are also promising. However, alterations of lifestyles may also provide highly favorable results in decreasing the amount of AGE produced and consumed by the body.

Diabetes and the complication of diabetic retinopathy are gradually on the rise and are widespread. Another disease that is nearly as widespread and also equally relevant in scientific study is Alzheimer's disease. Recent studies indicate that there may be a link between the two and the factors that are known to impact one of those diseases, such as AGEs, also have effects on the other [25]. Of organs that may exhibit diabetic complications, the eye and its associated connections are one that are closest physically to the brain, and one long-term study on retinal health and cognitive dysfunction showed that 40% of patients with DR showed reduced cognition [26]. Future studies in relation to AGEs will not only focus on the properties of AGEs and their impact on diabetes and its complications, but also how other illnesses are impacted by them as well.

Author details

Rujman Khan, Xin Yee Ooi*, Matthew Parvus, Laura Valdez and Andrew Tsin
Department of Molecular Science, University of Texas Rio Grande Valley, Edinburg, Texas, USA

*Address all correspondence to: xinyee.ooi01@utrgv.edu

References

[1] Zong H, Ward M, Stitt AW. AGEs, RAGE, and diabetic retinopathy. Current Diabetes Reports. 2011;**11**(4):244-252

[2] Prasad K, Mishra M. AGE-RAGE stress, stressors, and antistressors in health and disease. International Journal of Angiology. 2018;**27**(1):1-12

[3] Shimizu F et al. Advanced glycation end-products induce basement membrane hypertrophy in endoneurial microvessels and disrupt the blood-nerve barrier by stimulating the release of TGF-β and vascular endothelial growth factor (VEGF) by pericytes. Diabetologia. 2011;**54**(6):1517-1526

[4] Stitt AW. AGEs and diabetic retinopathy. Investigative Ophthalmology and Visual Science. 2010;**51**(10):4867-4874

[5] Singh R, Barden A, Mori T, Beilin L. Advanced glycation end-products: A review. Diabetologia. 2001;**44**:129-146

[6] Carvalho VF, Florim LT, de O Barreto E, Torres RC, Batista MM, Amendoeria FC, et al. Inhibition of advanced glycation end products by aminoguanidine restores mast cell numbers and reactivity in alloxan-diabetic rats. European Journal of Pharmacology. 2011;**669**(1):43-148

[7] Radoff S, Vlassara H, Cerami A. Characterization of solubilized cell surface binding protein on macrophages specific for proteins modified nonenzymatically by advanced glycation end products. Archives of Biochemistry and Biophysics. 1988;**263**(2):418-423

[8] Ramasamy R, Yan SF, Herold K, Clynes R, Schmidt AM. Receptor for advanced glycation end products: Fundamental roles in the inflammatory response: Winding the way to the pathogenesis of endothelial dysfunction and atherosclerosis. Annals of the New York Academy of Sciences. 2008;**1126**(1):7-13

[9] Rübsam A et al. Role of inflammation in diabetic retinopathy. International Journal of Molecular Sciences. 2018;**19**(4):1-31. DOI: 10.3390/ijms19040942

[10] Roy S et al. Extracellular matrix, gap junctions, and retinal vascular homeostasis in diabetic retinopathy. Experimental Eye Research. 2015;**133**:58-68

[11] Ferland-Mccollough D et al. Pericytes, an overlooked player in vascular pathobiology. Pharmacology and Therapeutics. 2017;**171**:30-42

[12] Li C et al. Oxidative stress-related mechanisms and antioxidant therapy in diabetic retinopathy. Oxidative Medicine and Cellular Longevity. 2017;**2017**:15

[13] Striker LJ, Striker GE. Administration of AGEs in vivo induces extracellular matrix gene expression. Nephrology, Dialysis, Transplantation: Official Publication of the European Dialysis and Transplant Association-European Renal Association. 1996;**11**(Suppl 5):62-65

[14] Duh E et al. Diabetic retinopathy: Current understanding, mechanisms, and treatment strategies. JCI Insight. 2017;**2**(14):1-14. DOI: 10.1172/jci.insight.93751

[15] Hammes H-P. Aminoguanidine treatment inhibits the development of experimental diabetic retinopathy. Proceedings of the National Academy of Sciences of the United States of America. 1991;**88**(24):11555-11558

[16] Nowotny K, Schroter D, Schreiner M, Grune T. Dietary advanced

glycation end products and their relevance for human health. Ageing Research Reviews. 2018;**47**:55-66

[17] Turk Z, Mesic R, Benko B. Comparison of advanced glycation end products on haemoglobin (Hb-AGE) and haemoglobin A1c for the assessment of diabetic control. Clinica Chimica Acta. 1998;**277**(2):159-170

[18] Remor AP, de Matos FJ, Ghisoni K, et al. Differential effects of insulin on peripheral diabetes-related changes in mitochondrial bioenergetics: Involvement of advanced glycosylated end products. Biochimica et Biophysica Acta-Molecular Basis of Disease. 2011;**1812**(11):1460-1471

[19] Stewart MW. Treatment of diabetic retinopathy: Recent advances and unresolved challenges. World Journal of Diabetes. 2016;**7**(16):333-341

[20] Picard S et al. Aminoguanidine inhibits oxidative modification of low density lipoprotein protein and the subsequent increase in uptake by macrophage scavenger receptors. Proceedings of the National Academy of Sciences of the United States of America. 1992;**89**(15):6876-6880

[21] Hammes H-P et al. Diabetic retinopathy: Targeting vasoregression. Diabetes. 2011;**60**(1):9-16

[22] Fan K, Li S, Liu G, Yuan H, Ma L, Lu P. Tanshinone IIA inhibits high glucose-induced proliferation, migration and vascularization of human retinal endothelial cells. Molecular Medicine Reports. 2017;**16**(6):9023-9028

[23] Qian S, Qian Y, Huo W, Qian Q. Tanshinone IIa protects retinal endothelial cells against mitochondrial fission induced by methylglyoxal through glyoxalase 1. European Journal of Pharmacology. 2019;**857**:1-10. DOI: 10.1016/j.ejphar.2019.172419

[24] Cerami C et al. Tobacco smoke is a source of toxic reactive glycation products. Proceedings of the National Academy of Sciences of the United States of America. 1997;**94**(25):13915-13920

[25] Jash K, Gondaliya P, Kirave P, Kulkarni B, Sunkaria A, Kalia K. Cognitive dysfunction: A growing link between diabetes and Alzheimer's disease. Drug Development Research. 2019;**80**(5):1-21. DOI: 10.1002/ddr.21579

[26] Nunley K, Ryan C, Saxton J, Orchard T, Costacou T, Aizenstein H. Early development of proliferative retinopathy increases risk of cognitive dysfunction in middle-aged adults with type 1 diabetes (P5.032). Neurology. 2015;**84**(14):1-5

Chapter 2

Deficient Autophagy Contributes to the Development of Diabetic Retinopathy

Jacqueline M. Lopes de Faria and Marcella Neves Dátilo

Abstract

Autophagy is a self-degradation process essential to maintain intracellular homeostasis and cell survival, controlling elimination of pathogens, damage to organelles, and nutrient recycling to generate energy. Alterations in autophagic flux have been reported in the mechanisms of several diseases such as neurodegenerative diseases, cancer, diabetes mellitus, and its associated complications. Diabetic retinopathy (DR) is a microvascular complication of diabetes, affecting nearly 30% of diabetic patients. Several pathways are triggered and repressed in the development of DR, and autophagy showed to be relevant in the pathogenesis of this devastating complication. In this chapter, autophagy's involvement in the development and progression of DR will be discussed, mainly in retinal pigmented epithelial cells and retinal microvascular endothelial cells, as well as in Müller cells—the more prominent retinal glial cell.

Keywords: retina, diabetic retinopathy, autophagy, ARPE-19, endothelial cell, Müller cell

1. Introduction

Autophagy (from Greek, meaning "self-eating") refers to a highly conserved process in eukaryotic cells, which coordinates the degradation of intracellular components and nutrient recycling. This process is essential for cellular homeostasis, survival, and differentiation. In basal conditions, the autophagic process happens in low levels to maintain cellular homeostasis. However, in such conditions as low levels of adenosine triphosphate (ATP) or depletion of essential amino acids and glucose, autophagic flux can increase to generate energy and raise basal levels. More recently, the understanding of this process has gained attention due to its pivotal role in cellular physiology and a variety of diseases from cancer, chronic degenerative diseases, and immune diseases (**Table 1**).

Autophagy is a primary cell response to stress and can be induced by starvation, endoplasmic reticulum (ER) stress, hypoxia, cytotoxicity, and infection (**Figure 1**). Sensation, initiation, and regulation of the autophagy–lysosomal pathway is controlled by the heterotrimeric serine/threonine kinase AMP (AMPK) and rapamycin complex 1 (mTORC1), either triggering or repressing autophagy and mitophagy. Unc-51-like kinase 1 (ULK1) is a primary initiating protein, as is mTORC1-supressed transcription factor EB (TFEB), which coordinates the synthesis of

Gene	Disease	References
GBA1[1], TMEM230[2]	Parkinson's disease	Schapira, 2015; Kim et al, 2017
PS1[3], APP[4]	Alzheimer's disease	Lee et al, 2010; Reddy et al, 2018
PTPN2[5]	Type 1 diabetes, juvenile arthritis	Scharl et al, 2012
ERBB2[6], FANC[7] genes	Breast Cancer	Vega-Rubin-de-Cellis et al, 2018; Sumpter et al, 2016
GPR65[8]	Inflammatory bowel disease	Lassen et al, 2016

Table 1.
In this table, some examples of genetic diseases associated with autophagic impairment [1–8].

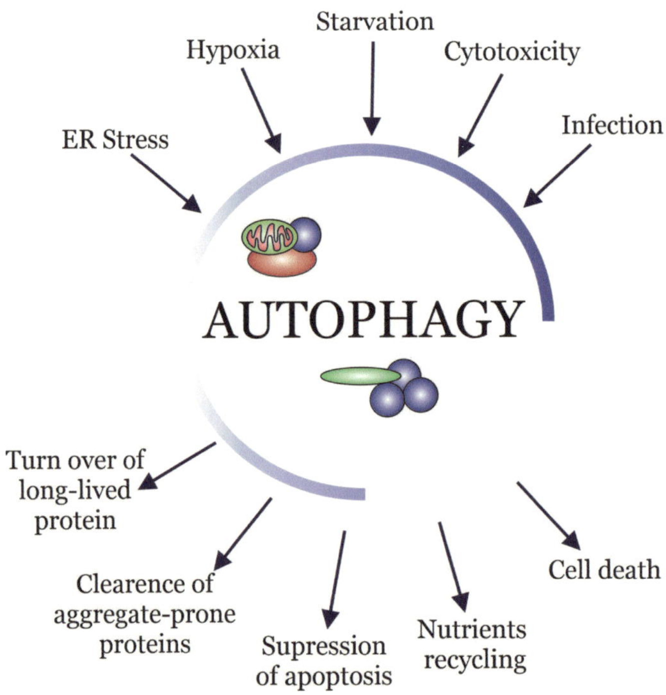

Figure 1.
Several cellular sensors regulate autophagic flux to maintain homeostasis.

lysosomes and other essential proteins maintaining the autophagic flux [9–12]. In addition, sirtuin-1—a class III deacetylase dependent on nicotinamide adenine dinucleotide (NAD+)—becomes a positive autophagy regulator, since it may also be considered a cellular sensor [13].

This process is mainly regulated at a post-translational level, increasing mRNA expression of autophagy genes [14]. Under stress conditions, TFEB is translocated from cytosol to the nucleus, activating transcription of ATG genes and coordinating upregulation of the entire autophagy–lysosomal pathway [15].

Autophagy can be constitutive or inducible, rapidly adjusting to alterations within the internal and external environment of the cells. Autophagy serves as a housekeeping system, demonstrated by animal models deficient in autophagy-related genes (ATG). For example, deletion of specific neurons of ATG7 or 5 genes leads to postnatal neurodegeneration [16, 17].

Intrinsically, cellular sensors detect changes in levels of glucose, cytosolic Ca^{++}, reactive oxygen species (ROS), and metabolic intermediates. Therefore, a decrease in glucose availability or impairment of mitochondrial respiration-compromising ATP production leads to an increase in the AMP/ADP ratio, activating the AMPK α subunit [10].

An example of extrinsic sensing occurs via drug-targetable mechanisms at the plasma membrane level. Tyrosine kinase receptors converge on mTOR, AMPK, or Beclin-1-Vps complex by modulating autophagy following growth factors [18, 19]. Even G-protein-coupled receptors (GPCRs) control autophagy via intracellular pathways that similarly modulate AMPK and mTOR [20–22].

This discussion includes a short overview of the more common types of autophagy and will highlight the role of autophagy in retinal diseases, with special attention to diabetic retinopathy.

2. Types of autophagy

There are three forms of autophagy previously described in the literature: macroautophagy, chaperone-mediated autophagy, and microautophagy (**Figure 2**).

2.1 Macroautophagy

Usually known as autophagy, this intracellular pathway includes cytosolic components such as proteins, lipids, organelles, and parts of the nucleus [23, 24]. Autophagy was first described by Christian du Duve 50 years ago and has been highly preserved across the species. From beginning to end, the whole process is controlled by the ATG protein family, and more than 35 genes have been identified to orchestrate the process [25].

Autophagosome formation is the hallmark of this process. The well-coordinated process begins with an initiation phase, when ULK1 kinase forms a complex with ATG13, ATG10, and FIP200 (known as RB1CC1) at a specific cell site located in the perivacuolar region known as the phagophore assembly site (PAS). ULK1 kinase activity triggers the formation of the phosphoinositide 3-kinase (PI3K) complex, which favors the formation of phosphatidylinositol 3-phosphate, initiating the nucleation phase [26]. Ubiquitin-like conjugation systems are then activated, catalyzed by ATG7. ATG12 is conjugated to ATG5, then phosphatidylethanolamine to microtubule-associated protein 1A/1B-light chain 3 (LC3) through ATG7 kinase, forming an autophagosome bound to LC3 (also called LC3-II) [27, 28]. The late stage of autophagy is controlled by molecules that regulate maturation of the autophagosome, fusion with lysosomes, acidification of the inside compartment of the autophagosome components, and recycling of metabolites from the lysosomal compartment. This coordinated process—including a sequence of protein–protein and protein–lipid interaction—is a dynamic process, where the autophagosome formation, fusion to the lysosome, and digestion of the inside components occur in less than 10 minutes. Therefore, any sort of autophagy dysfunction (such as blockage of lysosomal fusion or lysosomal function impairment) may lead to accumulation of harmful damaged organelles and protein aggregates inside the cell [29] (**Figure 2**).

2.2 Chaperone-mediated autophagy

In chaperone-mediated autophagy, there is no reorganization of the lysosomal membrane. This selective autophagy is only described in mammals [30], which

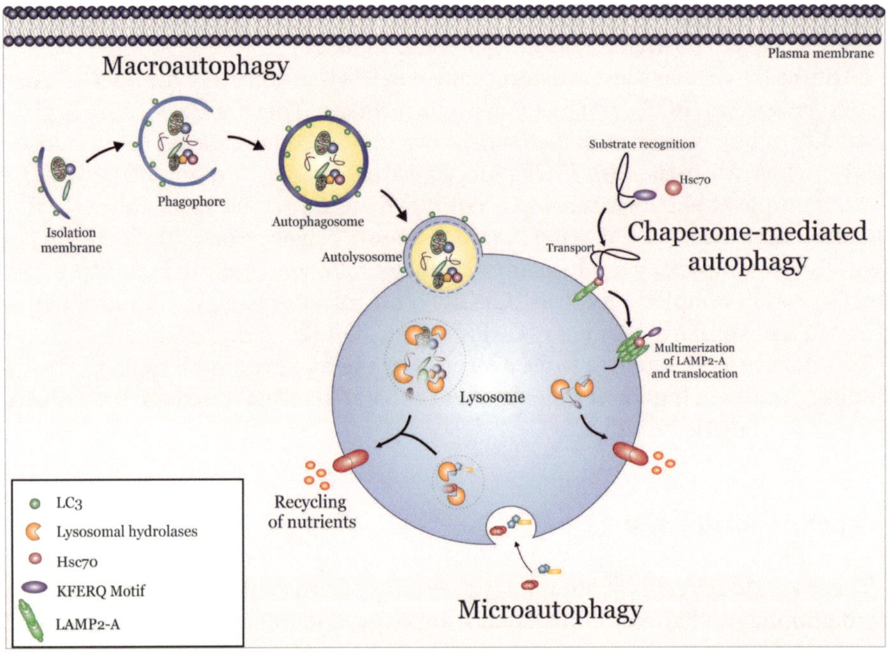

Figure 2.
Types of autophagy. (1) Macroautophagy: initiation of autophagy through isolation membrane, extension of membrane, and closure forming the autophagosome. Finally, the autophagosome merges with lysosome. Lysosomal hydrolases digest the contents to recycling nutrients. (2) Chaperone-mediated autophagy: identification of KFERQ-motif by Hsc70. Transportation of damage protein to lysosome. Recognition and multimerization of LAMP-2. Damage proteins are translocated to inside of the lysosome to suffer the action of lysosomal hydrolases. (3) Microautophagy: recognition and internalization of cytoplasmatic component.

mediates delivery of specific proteins to the lysosome. The distinction occurs because the cytosolic proteins need to be degraded by the presence of a pentapeptide amino acid sequence, KFERQ. This sequence permits recognition of the target protein by a family of chaperones and co-chaperones: the heat shock cognate, 70-kDa (Hsc70)—the most abundant in the family. After recognition of the KFERQ sequence, Hsc70 presents the unfolded proteins to the lysosome, one by one, where they are recognized by the transmembrane domain of lysosome-associated membrane protein type 2A (LAMP2-A). After this, the multimerization of LAMP2-A occurs, allowing transportation of the substrate into the lysosome for degradation. At the end of this process, the LAMP2-A complex is disassembled, and the chaperone Hsp70 is released to start a new cycle [31].

2.3 Microautophagy

Microautophagy is not well described in mammalian cells. However, recent evidence has shown that there is recognition and internalization of small cytoplasmatic components in late endosomes. This type of autophagy requires the chaperone Hsc70. However, the microautophagy process is independent of the unfolding of KFERQ and the multimerization of LAMP2-A [32, 33].

2.4 Role of autophagy in disease development

Since the primary function of autophagy is to eliminate harmful components from cells (aggregated proteins, damaged organelles, and pathogens), malfunctioning of this mechanism implicit in diseases—such as Huntington's and Parkinson's diseases [34, 35]—results in protein accumulation.

In physiological conditions, autophagy is involved in cellular homeostasis, as demonstrated in heart diseases, as seen in heart failure and ischemia–reperfusion injuries [36]. In the pancreas, autophagy is required to maintain function of β cells, revealing significance in the pathogenesis of diabetes. Alterations in autophagy have also been described in a more complex model in cancer research: it can suppress tumors but also helps the tumor adapt to metabolic stress in its late stages [37].

3. Diabetic retinopathy

Diabetes mellitus is a public health issue, estimated to affect about 500 million people by 2035 [38]. Nearly 30% of patients are likely to suffer from retinal microvascular complications and 10% may experience visual threatening due to macular edema or proliferative diabetic retinopathy [39, 40].

Multiple mechanisms are triggered under hyperglycemic conditions (hexosamine and polyol pathways [41], synthesis de novo of diacylglycerol-PKC [42, 43], low grade oxidative stress [44–46], inflammation [47–51], and advanced glycation end products [52, 53]). Although vascular changes are presumed to be the hallmarks of DR, abnormalities in retinal function are detected in patients with diabetes who have good visual acuity [54–59].

The characteristics of retinal neurodegeneration are apoptosis of neuro cells and dysfunction of glial cells—mainly Müller cells [29, 50, 60]. In microvascular disease of diabetic retinopathy, both inner and outer blood retinal barrier break down [61].

3.1 Autophagy in diabetic retinopathy

Since their pioneering studies, Remé et al. —describing the presence of active autophagy in photoreceptors during hibernation with a decreased number of mitochondria and organelles compared to animals in non-hibernating conditions—observed an increased number of autophagosomes [62]. These data show the pivotal role of autophagy in the retina, degrading cellular components (such as mitochondria) during hibernation.

Implications of autophagy in retinal ganglion cells (RGCs) attracted interest as a potential tool for neuroprotection in glaucoma. The first evidence of the cytoprotective role of autophagy in RGCs was shown by Rodríguez-Muela et al. using autophagy-deficient mice, which displayed increased axonal damage following optic nerve transection (ONT) models of optic neuropathy [63–65].

3.2 Autophagy in blood retinal barriers and implications on diabetic retinopathy

The main function of the blood-retina barrier (BRB) is maintenance of retinal homeostasis, regulating the transport of blood stream molecules to provide an appropriate supply for the neuroretina and to protect neural tissue against harmful agents present in the blood. The BRB is formed by two types of barriers: the inner blood-retina barrier (iBRB) and the outer blood-retina barrier (oBRB) [66].

Both outer and inner retinal barriers are affected by the toxic metabolic effects of hyperglycemia [67]. Alterations in the iBRB are more studied than the oBRB among the mechanisms of development and progression of DR [68–70]. The appropriated function of autophagy flux is important for maintenance of cellular viability and confers stress tolerance in retinal cells under adverse conditions such as DR [71].

Retinal endothelial cells of microcirculation of the retina form the iBRB. This barrier selectively allows passage of molecules from systemic circulation to retinal tissue. As a constituent of this barrier, there are tight junctions and adherens junctions such as zonula occludens-1 (ZO-1), occludin, VE-cadherin, and N-cadherin [72]. Endothelial cells are warped by pericytes, which are highly specialized. Pericytes play an essential role in the structure and stability of the iBRB, coordinating angiogenesis and vascular remodeling [73, 74].

Few articles have highlighted the autophagic process in retinal endothelial cells under diabetic conditions [75, 76]. Exposure to high glucose leads to an increase in retinal endothelial cell apoptosis, and this mechanism is mediated by the enhancement of ROS production. This phenomenon is correlated with a reduction in the AMPK pathway [76], which is well described as a direct activator of ULK-1 in the autophagy process [77]. Reestablishing the level of AMPK using specific activators—such as AICAR or antioxidant treatment—is effective in the protection of endothelial retinal cells from damage caused by diabetic conditions [75, 76]. A recent study from Niu et al. described the importance of the protective properties of metformin on retinal endothelial cells and human umbilical vascular endothelial cells (HUVECs) via autophagy in diabetic conditions. In this work, the authors showed that there was an increased LC3 puncta formation, which is an indicative of autophagy, in retinal vascular endothelium from db/db (diabetic) mice compared with control (non-diabetic) mice. This is indicative that metformin protects the retinal microvascular cells by diminishing LC3 formation. To further understand this mechanism, HUVECs were exposed to high levels of glucose and treated with metformin, resulting in a clear increase of LC3 formation. In HUVECs transfected with sh-PRKAA1/2 (AMP catalytic subunit), the protective effect of metformin was abrogated, indicating that metformin acts via AMPK activation [78] and improving autophagy in these cells.

The oBRB is a monolayer formed by retinal pigment epithelial cell layer that separates the neuro retina from choriocapillaris. Impairment of this barrier is implicated in diabetic retinopathy development [79–81]. The major functions of the oBRB are to provide glucose, fatty acids, and retinol to photoreceptors from choriocapillaris and reisomerise all-trans-retinal in 11-cis-retinal after photon absorption of the photoreceptor [66, 82, 83]. Therefore, any disturbance in this structure may have detrimental effects on the retina. A number of sight-threatening diseases display RPR dysfunction, such as age-related macular degeneration, proliferative vitreoretinopathy, and diabetic retinopathy [84].

It is well described in the literature that human retinal pigmented epithelial (RPE) immortalized cells (ARPE-19) exposed to high concentrations of glucose present molecular changes, including a decrease of proliferation, an increase in oxidative stress mediated by ROS production, and augmented lipid droplets and inflammation [85–88]. These alterations can activate or repress the autophagic flux in RPE cells. Studies have shown that, until 48 hours of exposure to high glucose levels, ARPE-19 cells present an increase in lipid droplets, which can contribute to ROS production [71, 85, 89]. This increase in ROS production can initiate autophagy, enhancing the numbers of autophagosomes, increasing conversion of LC3-I to LC3-II, and decreasing levels of p62/SQSTM1 as a defense mechanism against damage caused by high glucose. However, Chen et al. found that an increase in autophagic flux promoted by high glucose cannot be maintained long-term. After 7 days in high glucose, ARPE-19 presented impairment in the degradation of p62/SQSTM1 and an increase in apoptotic cells. These findings indicated that autophagy was the first defense against oxidative stress in high-glucose conditions. In the long-term, this protective pathway became saturated and inefficient, thus contributing to RPE degeneration in DR [87].

Zhang et al. have shown that high glucose concentrations can attenuate the PINK1 and parkin pathways involved in controlling cellular mitophagy. Downregulation of mitophagy can lead to an increase in cellular stress levels because the biogenesis of mitochondria becomes compromised [90].

The role of autophagy in retinal diabetic complications is not simply a matter of inhibiting its initiation or progression. Inhibition of autophagy in ARPE-19 during its initial phase with 3-methyladenine (3-MA) or during the fusion of autophagosome and lysosome using bafilomycin aggravates oxidative stress and exacerbates secretion of the pro-inflammatory interleukin-1β promoted by high glucose [88]. The appropriated autophagic process is important as a mechanism of cell homeostasis in diabetic conditions.

3.3 Autophagy in Müller glial cells and implications in diabetic retinopathy pathogenesis

Müller cells are the predominant glial cell in the retina. Its unique morphology allows the Müller cell to directly interact with neighboring neural and vascular cells, expanding through the entire retina from the inner limiting membrane to the photoreceptor layer. Müller cells are closely related with vitreous, blood vessels, and sub retinal space. Each Müller cell interacts with one cone and 10 rods [91]. This configuration of Müller cells inside the retina explains the diversity of its function, responsible for the metabolic, functional, and structural support of the retina [92].

There are several functions attributed to Müller cells, such as the release of trophic factors [93, 94], neurotransmitter recycling [95], and phagocytosis of external photoreceptor segments [96, 97]. Müller cells, depending upon the stimulus (trauma, vascular, or metabolic), may react with phenotype changes called gliosis, which consist in adaptive morphological, biochemical, and physiological alterations. Among the more interesting biochemical changes in Müller cells are increased vascular endothelial growth factor (VEGF) [98] and glial fibrillary acidic protein (GFAP) production, both with pro-angiogenic and pro-inflammatory effects. Massive VEGF release is present in the proliferative stages of DR and diabetic macular edema, representing a major therapeutic target for pharmacological treatment of these devastating complications.

There are few studies showing the effects of high glucose on autophagy in retinal Müller cells. Devi et al. described the implications of autophagy dysfunction in the mechanisms of DR [99]. In their study, Müller cells exposed to high glucose conditions for 5 days displayed an increase of autophagosome and mitophagosome in the cytosol, suggesting high glucose conditions activated the autophagy process. Despite activation of the protective process (autophagy), they observed an association with an increased proapoptotic caspase-3, leading to programmed cell death. This scenario elucidates that diabetic conditions induce activation of autophagy followed by dysfunction, leading to cellular death.

In the previously published work addressing the mechanism by which Müller cells exposed to high glucose release high amounts of VEFG and trigger increased apoptosis, it was shown that the autophagic process was defective in Müller cells among diabetic conditions. In cells exposed to high glucose, autophagy markers—both early Beclin and late LC3-I and LC3-II—were increased, but p62/SQSTM1 accumulated in the cytosol compartment of Müller cells, accompanied by an increased apoptotic rate. To further understand how p62/SQSTM1 could modulate the autophagy and apoptosis in Müller cells exposed to high glucose, p62/SQSTM1 was suppressed. In this condition, there was less endoplasmic reticulum stress, lowering the interaction with caspase-8 and, by extension, less apoptosis. The presence of rapamycin, an mTOR blocker, triggered the formation of autophagosome and ameliorated the degradation of p62/SQSTM1. Rapamycin showed to improve proteolytic activity of the lysosome, reducing the release of VEGF. Corresponding findings were also demonstrated in models using diabetic animals. In the retinas of diabetic rats, there was a significant increase in p62/SQSTM1 accumulation, particularly in cells located in the inner nuclear layer [29]. Lysosomal impairment and autophagic flux dysfunction are early indicators of the pathogenesis of DR.

4. Conclusion

Diabetic retinopathy is a neurodegenerative disease presenting vascular changes in its late stages. Multiple factors are associated with the development and progression of DR. Recently, better understanding at cellular and molecular levels of its process has been identified through the pathways and intracellular signaling involved in cells exposed to diabetic conditions. This has allowed identification of new therapeutic approaches. Recent concepts of this disease have been analyzed here, with special focus on the process of autophagy using experimental models in different retinal cells targeted by hyperglycemia in the developmental stages of the disease.

Author details

Jacqueline M. Lopes de Faria* and Marcella Neves Dátilo
Faculty of Medical Sciences, State University of Campinas, São Paulo, Brazil

*Address all correspondence to: lopesdefariajm@gmail.com

References

[1] Schapira AHV. Glucocerebrosidase and parkinson disease: Recent advances. Molecular and Cellular Neurosciences. 2015;**66**:37-42. DOI: 10.1016/j.mcn.2015.03.013

[2] Kim MJ, Deng H-X, Wong YC, Siddique T, Krainc D. The Parkinson's disease-linked protein TMEM230 is required for Rab8a-mediated secretory vesicle trafficking and retromer trafficking. Human Molecular Genetics. 2017;**26**(4):729-741. DOI: 10.1093/hmg/ddw413

[3] Lee J-H, Yu WH, Kumar A, Lee S, Mohan PS, Peterhoff CM, et al. Lysosomal proteolysis and autophagy require Presenilin 1 and are disrupted by Alzheimer-related PS1 mutations. Cell. 2010;**141**(7):1146-1158. DOI: 10.1016/j.cell.2010.05.008

[4] Reddy PH, Yin X, Manczak M, Kumar S, Pradeepkiran JA, Vijayan M, et al. Mutant APP and amyloid beta-induced defective autophagy, mitophagy, mitochondrial structural and functional changes and synaptic damage in hippocampal neurons from Alzheimer's disease. Human Molecular Genetics. 2018;**27**(14):2502-2516. DOI: 10.1093/hmg/ddy154

[5] Scharl M, Wojtal KA, Becker HM, Fischbeck A, Frei P, Arikkat J, et al. Protein tyrosine phosphatase nonreceptor type 2 regulates Autophagosome formation in human intestinal cells. Inflammatory Bowel Diseases. 2012;**18**(7):1287-1302. DOI: 10.1002/ibd.21891

[6] Vega-Rubín-de-Celis S, Zou Z, Fernández ÁF, Ci B, Kim M, Xiao G, et al. Increased autophagy blocks HER2-mediated breast tumorigenesis. Proceedings of the National Academy of Sciences. 2018;**115**(16):4176-4181. DOI: 10.1073/pnas.1717800115

[7] Sumpter R, Sirasanagandla S, Fernández ÁF, Wei Y, Dong X, Franco L, et al. Fanconi anemia proteins function in Mitophagy and immunity. Cell. 2016;**165**(4):867-881. DOI: 10.1016/j.cell.2016.04.006

[8] Lassen KG, McKenzie CI, Mari M, Murano T, Begun J, Baxt LA, et al. Genetic coding variant in GPR65 alters Lysosomal pH and links Lysosomal dysfunction with colitis risk. Immunity. 2016;**44**(6):1392-1405. DOI: 10.1016/j.immuni.2016.05.007

[9] Fernández ÁF, Sebti S, Wei Y, Zou Z, Shi M, McMillan KL, et al. Disruption of the beclin 1–BCL2 autophagy regulatory complex promotes longevity in mice. Nature. 2018;**558**(7708):136-140. DOI: 10.1038/s41586-018-0162-7

[10] Melendez A. Autophagy genes are essential for Dauer development and life-span extension in C. elegans. Science. 2003;**301**(5638):1387-1391. DOI: 10.1038/s41586-018-0162-7

[11] Hars ES, Qi H, Jin SV, Cai L, Hu C, Liu LF. Autophagy Regulates Ageing in C. elegans. Autophagy. 2007;**3**(2):93-95. DOI: 10.4161/auto.3636

[12] Hansen M, Chandra A, Mitic LL, Onken B, Driscoll M, Kenyon CA. Role for autophagy in the extension of lifespan by dietary restriction in C. elegans. PLoS Genetics. 2008;**4**(2):e24. DOI: 10.1371/journal.pgen.0040024.

[13] Juhasz G, Erdi B, Sass M, Neufeld TP. Atg7-dependent autophagy promotes neuronal health, stress tolerance, and longevity but is dispensable for metamorphosis in drosophila. Genes & Development. 2007;**21**(23):3061-3066. DOI: 10.1101/gad.1600707

[14] Feng Y, Yao Z, Klionsky DJ. How to control self-digestion: Transcriptional,

post-transcriptional, and post-translational regulation of autophagy. Trends in Cell Biology. 2015;**25**(6):354-363. DOI: 10.1016/j.tcb.2015.02.002

[15] Sardiello M, Palmieri M, di Ronza A, Medina DL, Valenza M, Gennarino VA, et al. A gene network regulating Lysosomal biogenesis and function. Science. 2009;**325**(5939):473-477. DOI: 10.1126/science.1174447

[16] Lipinski MM, Zheng B, Lu T, Yan Z, Py BF, Ng A, et al. Genome-wide analysis reveals mechanisms modulating autophagy in normal brain aging and in Alzheimer's disease. Proceedings of the National Academy of Sciences. 2010;**107**(32):14164-14169. DOI: 10.1016/j.cellsig.2013.06.013

[17] Chen Y, Sawada O, Kohno H, Le YZ, Subauste C, Maeda T, et al. Autophagy protects the retina from light-induced degeneration. The Journal of Biological Chemistry. 2013;**288**(11):7506-7518. DOI: 10.1074/jbc.M112.439935

[18] Zhao J, Brault JJ, Schild A, Cao P, Sandri M, Schiaffino S, et al. FoxO3 coordinately activates protein degradation by the Autophagic/Lysosomal and proteasomal pathways in atrophying muscle cells. Cell Metabolism. 2007;**6**(6):472-483. DOI: 10.1016/j.cmet.2007.11.004

[19] Sarkis GJ, Ashcom JD, Hawdon JM, Jacobson LA. Decline in protease activities with age in the nematode caenorhabditis elegans. Mechanisms of Ageing and Development. 1988;**45**(3):191-201. DOI: 10.1016/0047-6374(88)90001-2

[20] Kuma A, Hatano M, Matsui M, Yamamoto A, Nakaya H, Yoshimori T, et al. The role of autophagy during the early neonatal starvation period. Nature. 2004;**432**(7020):1032-1036. DOI: 10.1038/nature03029

[21] Kapahi P, Kaeberlein M, Hansen M. Dietary restriction and lifespan: Lessons from invertebrate models. Ageing Research Reviews. 2017;**39**:3-14. DOI: 10.1016/j.arr.2016.12.005

[22] Mattison JA, Colman RJ, Beasley TM, Allison DB, Kemnitz JW, Roth GS, et al. Caloric restriction improves health and survival of rhesus monkeys. Nature Communications. 2017;**8**(1):14063. DOI: 10.1038/ncomms14063

[23] Boya P, Reggiori F, Codogno P. Emerging regulation and functions of autophagy. Nature Cell Biology. 2013;**15**(7):713-720. DOI: 10.1038/ncb2788

[24] Dou Z, Xu C, Donahue G, Shimi T, Pan JA, Zhu J, et al. Autophagy mediates degradation of nuclear lamina. Nature. 2015;**527**(7576):105-109. DOI: 10.1038/nature15548

[25] Ktistakis NT, Tooze SA. Digesting the expanding mechanisms of autophagy. Trends in Cell Biology. 2016;**26**(8):624-635. DOI: 10.1016/j.tcb.2016.03.006

[26] Bento CF, Renna M, Ghislat G, Puri C, Ashkenazi A, Vicinanza M, et al. Mammalian autophagy: How does it work? Annual Review of Biochemistry. 2016;**85**(1):685-713. DOI: 10.1146/annurev-biochem-060815-014556

[27] Choi AMK, Ryter SW, Levine B. Mechanisms of disease: Autophagy in human health and disease. The New England Journal of Medicine. 2013;**368**(7):651-662. DOI: 10.1056/NEJMra1205406

[28] Suzuki H, Osawa T, Fujioka Y, Noda NN. Structural biology of the core autophagy machinery. Current Opinion in Structural Biology. 2017;**43**:10-17. DOI: 10.1016/j.sbi.2016.09.010

[29] Lopes de Faria JM, Duarte DA, Montemurro C, Papadimitriou A, Consonni SR, Lopes de Faria JB. Defective autophagy in diabetic retinopathy. Investigative Ophthalmology & Visual Science. 2016;**57**(10):4356. DOI: 10.1167/iovs.16-19197

[30] Arias E, Cuervo AM. Chaperone-mediated autophagy in protein quality control. Current Opinion in Cell Biology. 2011;**23**(2):184-189. DOI: 10.1016/j.ceb.2010.10.009

[31] Orenstein SJ, Cuervo AM. Chaperone-mediated autophagy: Molecular mechanisms and physiological relevance. Seminars in Cell & Developmental Biology. 2010;**21**(7):719-726. DOI: 10.1074/jbc.R117.818237

[32] Sahu R, Kaushik S, Clement CC, Cannizzo ES, Scharf B, Follenzi A, et al. Microautophagy of cytosolic proteins by late endosomes. Developmental Cell. 2011;**20**(1):131-139. DOI: 10.1016/j.devcel.2010.12.003

[33] Tekirdag K, Cuervo AM. Chaperone-mediated autophagy and endosomal microautophagy: Jointed by a chaperone. The Journal of Biological Chemistry. 2018;**293**(15):5414-5424. DOI: 10.1074/jbc.R117.818237

[34] Moloudizargari M, Asghari MH, Ghobadi E, Fallah M, Rasouli S, Abdollahi M. Autophagy, its mechanisms and regulation: Implications in neurodegenerative diseases. Ageing Research Reviews. 2017;**40**:64-74. DOI: 10.1016/j.arr.2017.09.005

[35] Menzies FM, Fleming A, Caricasole A, Bento CF, Andrews SP, Ashkenazi A, et al. Autophagy and Neurodegeneration: Pathogenic mechanisms and therapeutic opportunities. Neuron. 2017;**93**(5):1015-1034. DOI: 10.1016/j.neuron.2017.01.022

[36] Lavandero S, Chiong M, Rothermel BA, Hill JA. Autophagy in cardiovascular biology. The Journal of Clinical Investigation. 2015;**125**(1):55-64. DOI: 10.1172/JCI73943

[37] Galluzzi L, Bravo-San Pedro JM, Kroemer G. Autophagy mediates tumor suppression via cellular senescence. Trends in Cell Biology. 2016;**26**(1):1-3. DOI: 10.1016/j.tcb.2015.11.001

[38] Wild S, Roglic G, Green A, Sicree R, King H. Global prevalence of diabetes: Estimates for the year 2000 and projections for 2030. Diabetes Care. 2004;**27**(5):1047-1053. DOI: 10.2337/diacare.27.5.1047

[39] Yau JWY, Rogers SL, Kawasaki R, Lamoureux EL, Kowalski JW, Bek T, et al. Global prevalence and major risk factors of diabetic retinopathy. Diabetes Care. 2012;**35**(3):556-564. DOI: 10.2337/dc11-1909

[40] Kempen JH, O'Colmain BJ, Leske MC, Haffner SM, Klein R, Moss SE, et al. The prevalence of diabetic retinopathy among adults in the United States. Archives of Ophthalmology. 2004;**122**(4):552-563. DOI: 10.1001/archopht.122.4.552

[41] Berrone E, Beltramo E, Solimine C, Ape AU, Porta M. Regulation of intracellular glucose and polyol pathway by thiamine and benfotiamine in vascular cells cultured in high glucose. The Journal of Biological Chemistry. 2006;**281**(14):9307-9313. DOI: 10.1074/jbc.M600418200

[42] Geraldes P, King GL. Activation of protein kinase C isoforms and its impact on diabetic complications. Circulation Research. 2010;**106**(8):1319-1331. DOI: 10.1161/CIRCRESAHA.110.217117

[43] Lee TS, Saltsman KA, Ohashi H, King GL. Activation of protein kinase C

by elevation of glucose concentration: Proposal for a mechanism in the development of diabetic vascular complications. Proceedings of the National Academy of Sciences. 2006;**86**(13):5141-5145. DOI: 10.1073/pnas.86.13.5141

[44] Wu M, Yiang G, Lai T, Li C. The oxidative stress and mitochondrial dysfunction during the pathogenesis of diabetic retinopathy. Oxidative Medicine and Cellular Longevity. 2018;**2018**:1-12. DOI: 10.1155/2018/3420187

[45] Rosales MAB, Silva KC, Duarte DA, Rossato FA, Lopes de Faria JB, Lopes de Faria JM. Endocytosis of tight junctions Caveolin Nitrosylation dependent is improved by cocoa via opioid receptor on RPE cells in diabetic conditions. Investigative Ophthalmology & Visual Science. 2014;**55**(9):6090. DOI: 10.1167/iovs.14-14234

[46] Brownlee M. The pathobiology of diabetic complications: A unifying mechanism. Diabetes. 2005;**54**(6):1615-1625. DOI: 10.3390/nu8090585

[47] Li J, Schmidt AM. Characterization and functional analysis of the promoter of RAGE, the receptor for advanced glycation end products. The Journal of Biological Chemistry. 1997;**272**(26):16498-16506. DOI: 10.1074/jbc.272.26.16498

[48] Rajagopal R, Bligard GW, Zhang S, Yin L, Lukasiewicz P, Semenkovich CF. Functional deficits precede structural lesions in mice with high-fat diet-induced diabetic retinopathy. Diabetes. 2016;**65**:1-35. DOI: 10.2337/db15-1255

[49] Shelton MD, Kern TS, Mieyal JJ. Glutaredoxin regulates nuclear factor κ-B and intercellular adhesion molecule in Müller cells: Model of diabetic retinopathy. The Journal of Biological Chemistry. 2007;**282**(17):12467-12474. DOI: 10.1074/jbc.M610863200

[50] Duarte DA, Papadimitriou A, Gilbert RE, Thai K, Zhang Y, Rosales MAB, et al. Conditioned medium from early-outgrowth bone marrow cells is retinal protective in experimental model of diabetes. PLoS One. 2016;**11**(2):e0147978. DOI: 10.1371/journal.pone.0147978

[51] Dátilo MN, Sant'Ana MR, Formigari GP, Rodrigues PB, de Moura LP, da Silva ASR, et al. Omega-3 from flaxseed oil protects obese mice against diabetic retinopathy through GPR120 receptor. Scientific Reports. 2018;**8**(1):14318. DOI: 10.1038/s41598-018-32553-5

[52] Genuth S, Sun W, Cleary P, Gao X, Sell DR, Lachin J, et al. Skin advanced glycation end products glucosepane and methylglyoxal hydroimidazolone are independently associated with long-term microvascular complication progression of type 1 diabetes. Diabetes. 2015;**64**(1):266-278. DOI: 10.1007/s00726-010-0773-2

[53] Treins C, Giorgetti-Peraldi S, Murdaca J, Van Obberghen E. Regulation of vascular endothelial growth factor expression by advanced Glycation end products. The Journal of Biological Chemistry. 2001;**276**(47):43836-43841. DOI: 10.1074/jbc.M106534200

[54] Hyvarärinen L, Laurinen P, Rovamo J. Contrast sensitivity in evaluation of visual impairment due to diabetes. Acta Ophthalmologica. 2009;**61**(1):94-101. DOI: 10.1111/j.1755-3768.1983.tb01399.x

[55] Sokol S, Moskowitz A, Skarf B, Evans R, Molitch M, Senior B. Contrast sensitivity in diabetics with and without background retinopathy. Archives of Ophthalmology. 1985;**103**(1):51-54. DOI: 10.1001/archopht.1985.01050010055018

[56] Hardy KJ, Lipton J, Scase MO, Foster DH, Scarpello JHB. Detection of colour vision abnormalities in uncomplicated type 1 diabetic patients with angiographically normal retinas. The British Journal of Ophthalmology. 1992;**76**(8):461-464. DOI: 10.1136/bjo.76.8.461

[57] Bresnick GH. Electroretinographic oscillatory potentials predict progression of diabetic retinopathy. Archives of Ophthalmology. 1984;**102**(9):1307. DOI: 10.1167/iovs.04-1409

[58] Lopes de Faria J, Katsumi O, Cagliero E, Nathan D, Hirose T. Neurovisual abnormalities preceding the retinopathy in patients with long-term type 1 diabetes mellitus. Graefe's Archive for Clinical and Experimental Ophthalmology. 2001;**239**(9):643-648. DOI: 10.1007/s004170100268

[59] Simó R, Hernández C. Neurodegeneration in the diabetic eye: New insights and therapeutic perspectives. Trends in Endocrinology and Metabolism. 2014;**25**(1):23-33. DOI: 10.1016/j.tem.2013.09.005

[60] Duarte DA, Rosales MAB, Papadimitriou A, Silva KC, Amancio VHO, Mendonça JN, et al. Polyphenol-enriched cocoa protects the diabetic retina from glial reaction through the sirtuin pathway. The Journal of Nutritional Biochemistry. 2015;**26**(1):64-74. DOI: 10.1016/j.jnutbio.2014.09.003

[61] Li PSH, Wong TH, Tang WWT, Lai JSM. Diabetic retinopathy. Hong Kong Practice. 2004;**26**(8):346-353. DOI: 10.1038/nrdp.2016.12

[62] Remé CE, Young RW. The effects of hibernation on cone visual cells in the ground squirrel. Investigative Ophthalmology and Visual Science. 1977;**16**(9):815-840

[63] Rodríguez-Muela N, Germain F, Mariño G, Fitze PS, Boya P. Autophagy promotes survival of retinal ganglion cells after optic nerve axotomy in mice. Cell Death and Differentiation. 2012;**19**(1):162-169. DOI: 10.1038/cdd.2011.88

[64] Rodríguez-Muela N, Boya P. Axonal damage, autophagy and neuronal survival. Autophagy. 2012;**8**(2):286-288. DOI: 10.4161/auto.8.2.18982

[65] Kurz T, Karlsson M, Brunk UT, Nilsson SE, Frennesson C. ARPE-19 retinal pigment epithelial cells are highly resistant to oxidative stress and exercise strict control over their lysosomal redox-active iron. Autophagy. 2009;**5**(4):494-501. DOI: 10.4161/auto.5.4.7961

[66] Cunha-Vaz J, Bernardes R, Lobo C. Blood-retinal barrier. European Journal of Ophthalmology. 2011;**21**(Suppl 6):3-9. DOI: 10.5301/EJO.2010.6049

[67] Di Rosa M, Distefano G, Gagliano C, Rusciano D, Malaguarnera L. Autophagy in diabetic retinopathy. Current Neuropharmacology. 2016;**14**(8):810-825. DOI: 10.2174/1570159X14666160321122900

[68] Rübsam A, Parikh S, Fort P. Role of inflammation in diabetic retinopathy. International Journal of Molecular Sciences. 2018;**19**(4):942. DOI: 10.3390/ijms19040942

[69] Díaz-Coránguez M, Ramos C, Antonetti DA. The inner blood-retinal barrier: Cellular basis and development. Vision Research. 2017;**139**:123-137. DOI: 10.1016/j.visres.2017.05.009

[70] Gardner TW, Antonetti DA, Barber AJ, LaNoue KF, Levison SW. Diabetic retinopathy: More than meets the eye. Survey of Ophthalmology. 2002;**47**:S253-S262. DOI: 10.1016/S0039-6257(02)00387-9

[71] Huang C, Lu H, Xu J, Yu H, Wang X, Zhang X. Protective roles of autophagy in retinal pigment epithelium under high glucose condition via regulating PINK1/Parkin pathway and BNIP3L. Biological Research. 2018;**51**(1):22. DOI: 10.1186/s40659-018-0169-4

[72] Daruich A, Matet A, Moulin A, Kowalczuk L, Nicolas M, Sellam A, et al. Mechanisms of macular edema: Beyond the surface. Progress in Retinal and Eye Research. 2018;**63**:20-68. DOI: 10.1016/j.preteyeres.2017.10.006

[73] Gerhardt H, Betsholtz C. Endothelial-pericyte interactions in angiogenesis. Cell and Tissue Research. 2003;**314**(1):15-23. Available from: http://link.springer.com/10.1007/s00441-003-0745-x

[74] Park DY, Lee J, Kim J, Kim K, Hong S, Han S, et al. Plastic roles of pericytes in the blood–retinal barrier. Nature Communications. 2017;**8**(1):15296. DOI: 10.1007/s00441-003-0745-x

[75] Mao XB, You ZP, Wu C, Huang J. Potential suppression of the high glucose and insulin-induced retinal neovascularization by Sirtuin 3 in the human retinal endothelial cells. Biochemical and Biophysical Research Communications. 2017;**482**(2):341-345. DOI: 10.1016/j.bbrc.2016.11.065

[76] Li J, Yu S, Ying J, Shi T, Wang P. Resveratrol prevents ROS-induced apoptosis in high glucose-treated retinal capillary endothelial cells via the activation of AMPK/Sirt1/PGC-1 α pathway. Oxidative Medicine and Cellular Longevity. 2017;**2017**:1-10. DOI: 10.1155/2017/7584691

[77] Kim J, Kundu M, Viollet B, Guan K-L. AMPK and mTOR regulate autophagy through direct phosphorylation of Ulk1. Nature Cell Biology. 2011;**13**(2):132-141. DOI: 10.1038/ncb2152

[78] Niu C, Chen Z, Kim KT, Sun J, Xue M, Chen G, et al. Metformin alleviates hyperglycemia-induced endothelial impairment by downregulating autophagy via the hedgehog pathway. Autophagy. 2019;**15**(5):843-870. DOI: 10.1080/15548627.2019.1569913

[79] Simó R, Villarroel M, Corraliza L, Hernández C, Garcia-Ramírez M. The retinal pigment epithelium: Something more than a constituent of the blood-retinal barrier-implications for the pathogenesis of diabetic retinopathy. Journal of Biomedicine and Biotechnology. 2010;**2010**:190724. DOI: 10.1155/2010/190724

[80] Xu H-Z, Le Y-Z. Significance of outer blood–retina barrier breakdown in diabetes and ischemia. Investigative Ophthalmology & Visual Science. 2011;**52**(5):2160. DOI: 10.1167/iovs.10-6518

[81] Xia T, Rizzolo LJ. Effects of diabetic retinopathy on the barrier functions of the retinal pigment epithelium. Vision Research. 2017;**139**:72-81. DOI: 10.1016/j.visres.2017.02.006

[82] Strauss O. The retinal pigment epithelium in visual function. Physiological Reviews. 2005;**85**(3):845-881. DOI: 10.1152/physrev.00021.2004

[83] Amram B, Cohen-Tayar Y, David A, Ashery-Padan R. The retinal pigmented epithelium – From basic developmental biology research to translational approaches. The International Journal of Developmental Biology. 2017;**61**(3-4-5):225-234. DOI: 10.1387/ijdb.160393ra

[84] Vinores SA, Gadegbeku C, Campochiaro PA, Green WR. Immunohistochemical localization of blood-retinal barrier breakdown in

human diabetics. The American Journal of Pathology. 1989;**134**(2):231-235

[85] Zhang W, Song J, Zhang Y, Ma Y, Yang J, He G, et al. Intermittent high glucose-induced oxidative stress modulates retinal pigmented epithelial cell autophagy and promotes cell survival via increased HMGB1. BMC Ophthalmology. 2018;**18**(1):192. DOI: 10.1016/j.biopha.2019.01.034

[86] Boya P, Esteban-Martínez L, Serrano-Puebla A, Gómez-Sintes R, Villarejo-Zori B. Autophagy in the eye: Development, degeneration, and aging. Progress in Retinal and Eye Research. 2016;**55**:206-245. DOI: 10.1016/j.preteyeres.2016.08.001

[87] Chen Q, Tang L, Xin G, Li S, Ma L, Xu Y, et al. Oxidative stress mediated by lipid metabolism contributes to high glucose-induced senescence in retinal pigment epithelium. Free Radical Biology & Medicine. 2019;**130**:48-58. DOI: 10.1016/j.freeradbiomed.2018.10.419

[88] Shi H, Zhang Z, Wang X, Li R, Hou W, Bi W, et al. Inhibition of autophagy induces IL-1β release from ARPE-19 cells via ROS mediated NLRP3 inflammasome activation under high glucose stress. Biochemical and Biophysical Research Communications. 2015;**463**(4):1071-1076. DOI: 10.1016/j.bbrc.2015.06.060

[89] Filomeni G, De Zio D, Cecconi F. Oxidative stress and autophagy: The clash between damage and metabolic needs. Cell Death and Differentiation. 2015;**22**(3):377-388. DOI: 10.1038/cdd.2014.150

[90] Zhang Y, Xi X, Mei Y, Zhao X, Zhou L, Ma M, et al. High-glucose induces retinal pigment epithelium mitochondrial pathways of apoptosis and inhibits mitophagy by regulating ROS/PINK1/Parkin signal pathway. Biomedicine & Pharmacotherapy. 2019;**111**:1315-1325. DOI: 10.1016/j.biopha.2019.01.034

[91] Reichenbach A, Bringmann A. Müller Cells in the Healthy and Diseased Retina. Müller Cells in the Healthy and Diseased Retina. New York, NY: Springer New York; 2010. DOI: 10.1007/978-1-4419-1672-3

[92] Vecino E, Rodriguez FD, Ruzafa N, Pereiro X, Sharma SC. Glia–neuron interactions in the mammalian retina. Progress in Retinal and Eye Research. 2016;**51**:1-40. DOI: 10.1016/j.preteyeres.2015.06.003

[93] Pow DV, Crook DK. Direct immunocytochemical evidence for the transfer of glutamine from glial cells to neurons: Use of specific antibodies directed against thed-stereoisomers of glutamate and glutamine. Neuroscience. 1996;**70**(1):295-302. DOI: 10.1016/0306-4522(95)00363-N

[94] Powell C, Grant AR, Cornblath E, Goldman D. Analysis of DNA methylation reveals a partial reprogramming of the Muller glia genome during retina regeneration. Proceedings of the National Academy of Sciences. 2013;**110**(49):19814-19819. DOI: 10.1073/pnas.1312009110

[95] Schütte M, Werner P. Redistribution of glutathione in the ischemic rat retina. Neuroscience Letters. 1998;**246**(1):53-56. DOI: 10.1016/S0304-3940(98)00229-8

[96] Long KO, Fisher SK, Fariss RN, Anderson DH. Disc shedding and autophagy in the cone-dominant ground squirrel retina. Experimental Eye Research. 1986;**43**(2):193-205. DOI: 10.1016/S0014-4835(86)80087-2

[97] Wang JS, Kefalov VJ. The cone-specific visual cycle. Progress in Retinal and Eye Research. 2011;**30**(2):115-128. DOI: 10.1016/j.preteyeres.2010.11.001

[98] Bai Y, Ma J, Guo J, Wang J, Zhu M, Chen Y, et al. Müller cell-derived VEGF is a significant contributor to retinal neovascularization. The Journal of Pathology. 2009;**219**(4):446-454. DOI: 10.1002/path.2611

[99] Devi TS, Lee I, Hüttemann M, Kumar A, Nantwi KD, Singh LP. TXNIP links innate host defense mechanisms to oxidative stress and inflammation in retinal Muller glia under chronic hyperglycemia: Implications for diabetic retinopathy. Experimental Diabetes Research. 2012;**2012**:1-19. DOI: 10.1155/2012/438238

Chapter 3

Diabetic Vitrectomy

Ogugua N. Okonkwo

Abstract

Diabetic retinopathy (DR) in its advanced stage is a leading cause of blindness and visual impairment. Despite efforts at early detection of DR, disease monitoring, and medical therapy, significant proportions of people living with diabetes still progress to develop the advanced proliferative disease, which is characterized by neovascularization, actively proliferating fibrovascular membranes, and retinal traction. The surgical removal of this proliferating tissue and the treatment of the retinal ischemic drive can be very rewarding, providing significant stability of the retina and in several cases improved retinal anatomy and vision. Diabetic vitrectomy comprises a broad range of surgical techniques and maneuvers, which offer the surgeon and patient opportunity to reverse deranged vitreoretinal anatomy and improve or stabilizes vision. Advances in vitreoretinal technology have contributed greatly to more recent improved outcomes; it is expected that future advances will offer even more benefit.

Keywords: diabetic retinopathy, vitreous hemorrhage, proliferative diabetic retinopathy, tractional retinal detachment, macular edema, vitrectomy

1. Introduction

Global estimates of diabetes have been on the rise [1]. Diabetic retinopathy (DR) is a leading cause of blindness among the working age group, with increasing numbers of persons being affected worldwide [2, 3]. It is a microvascular complication of diabetes which progresses to advanced disease in several cases. It is a global concern as indicated by a recent review published in Lancet [4]. The microvascular complications of diabetes result in macular leakage or exudation and vasoproliferative retinal disease, which are the hallmarks of advanced DR. Despite treatment of earlier stages of DR with medical therapy, which include intravitreal injection of anti-vascular endothelial growth factor (VEGF), intravitreal injection of steroids, and retinal laser photocoagulation, several eyes will progress to require surgical treatment [5–8].

Surgical treatment for the advanced complications of DR can range from more straightforward cases involving the removal of a non-clearing vitreous hemorrhage from an eye in which vitreous separation has already occurred, to more complicated surgical techniques such as in dealing with a combined tractional and rhegmatogenous retinal detachment (TRD/RRD) or tractional retinal detachment (TRD) involving the macula [9, 10]. The preoperative considerations, intraoperative techniques, and the postoperative outcome, including the complications of surgery, could vary considerably, depending on the risk factors and complexity of the vitreoretinal presentation associated with each case. Therefore surgical planning should be done on a case-by-case basis.

Furthermore, in recent times, there have been significant improvements in preoperative care and evaluation, and intraoperative surgical technique, including the administration of preoperative intravitreal pharmacotherapy, development of small-gauge transconjunctival instrumentation [11–13], and availability of multifunctional vitrectomy probes with high cut rates [14]. These advances have made surgical outcome more predictable and have resulted in an expansion of the indication for vitrectomy in the management of the tractional complications seen in DR. This review will focus on highlighting the indications, pathophysiology and principles of surgery, preoperative considerations, intraoperative surgical techniques, and outcome of diabetic vitrectomy in contemporary times.

2. Indications for surgery

The indications for vitrectomy in advanced DR have increased over the years from the situation in the early years of diabetic vitrectomy, when surgery was used for removing non-clearing vitreous hemorrhage. The first vitrectomy performed by Machemer was for the removal of non-clearing vitreous hemorrhage in a patient living with diabetes, and suffering from proliferative diabetic retinopathy (PDR) [15]. The Diabetic Retinopathy Vitrectomy Study (DRVS) was the first randomized, large series study evaluating the outcome of early versus deferral of vitrectomy in eyes with vitreous hemorrhage secondary to advanced DR [16]. It highlighted the benefit of early vitrectomy especially in type 1 diabetics with more severe disease. The DRVS also demonstrated that the benefit of surgery was maintained over a 4-year study period. Since then, the indications for diabetic vitrectomy (DV) are now known to include non-clearing vitreous hemorrhage, TRD, combined RRD/TRD, vitreomacular traction, traction-induced diabetic macular edema (DME), rubeosis iridis, and macular distortion (including dragging of the macula), to mention a few [17–21].

1. Vitreous hemorrhage (VH): vitrectomy for vitreous hemorrhage removal, in several studies, remains the most common indication for diabetic vitrectomy [20, 22, 23]. The scope of this will depend on the surgeon's personal experience, state of the fellow eye, previous retinal laser, recurrence of VH, and systemic control of glycemic levels. Non-clearing vitreous hemorrhage cases with complete separation of the posterior hyaloid are rather uncommon and the vitreous can be easily removed with expectation of improved vision in a majority of eyes. Vitrectomy for a case in which prior retinal laser photocoagulation has been applied also tends to progress quite well as the prior laser would have reduced the activity of the retinopathy, treated the retinal ischemia, and slowed the momentum of the disease. Moreover, in eyes with prior preoperative retinal laser, the occurrence of iatrogenic breaks within the areas of retinal laser scars prevents progression to retinal detachment. VH can at times be associated with more severe proliferative retinal disease such as a macula involving TRD. In this case both VH and TRD are indications for surgery and eventual visual outcome will be affected by the occurrence of TRD. This situation can be identified using a preoperative B scan ultrasound, which will reveal the TRD.

2. Retinal traction involving the macula can be an important indication for vitrectomy. This can occur as a result of an epiretinal membrane (ERM), TRD, TRD/RRD and vitreomacular traction (VMT). Fibrovascular proliferation (FVP) in the sub-hyaloid space is responsible for the retinal traction, which could initially occur in an extra macular site, and then progress to involve the macular area. Also, TRD could develop primarily in the macula and have an early impact on vision.

Surgery is indicated when the traction occurs in the macula or if there is obvious progression of an extra macular TRD towards the macula. In some cases the retinal traction is significant and creates a retinal tear. This adds a rhegmatogenous component to the already existing TRD. In combined TRD/RRD, progression to involve the macula could be rapid, and early surgery is advised.

In these situations of significant traction involving the macula or threatening the macula, surgery is indicated to relieve the traction and reattach the retina or to prevent progression of TRD to the macula. However, there are several cases in which extra macular TRD remains stable after adequate panretinal laser photocoagulation (PRP) and good control of systemic parameters have been achieved. Such cases can be observed since there is no progression.

In one review comparing African-Americans with Caucasians requiring diabetic vitrectomy, patients of African-American descent were found to be more likely to have TRD/RRD than Caucasians, and it was concluded that African-Americans might have a greater risk of developing this advanced complication [24]. In the light of this, African-Americans and others at increased risk could benefit from earlier vitrectomy, before the onset of vision damaging advanced tractional complications.

3. Persistent retinal neovascularization despite adequate laser PRP may result in recurrent VH and requires surgical removal of the vitreous scaffolding on which such neovascularization would progress. In such cases, adequate retinal laser fails to cause a complete regression of neovascularization. The vascular tuft invades the vitreous scaffold and forms neovascular pegs. This vitreous attachment to the neovascular peg has to be removed to prevent the recurrent VH, which recurs whenever there is significant vitreous traction on the neovascular tuft.

4. Severe FVP, especially if associated with significant traction involving or threatening the macula, or if obscuring the macula, may require surgical removal. In some instances, FVP occurs in the retina periphery and may be associated with proliferation extending from sclerotomy sites. This was more common in the era of large sclerotomies using the 20-gauge vitrectomy systems. Residual postoperative peripheral vitreous and significant untreated ischemia in the peripheral retina using either endoretinal laser photocoagulation or cryotherapy predispose to the formation of this complication better known as anterior hyaloidal fibrovascular proliferation (AHFVP) [25]. This is a known complication of diabetic vitrectomy which has also been reported to occur after cataract surgery in poorly controlled diabetic patients [25, 26].

Other indications for diabetic vitrectomy include macular ectopia and rubeotic glaucoma.

3. Preoperative systemic considerations

Diabetes is a multisystem disease. The presence of DR suggests microvascular affectation, which may include an effect on the microvasculature in other organs, especially the kidney resulting in diabetic nephropathy. Advanced retinopathy requiring surgery has been found to be associated with reduced life expectancy [27]. Also patients with diabetic macular edema have been noted to have a higher incidence of cerebrovascular accidents and myocardial infarcts [28].

As the patient for diabetic vitrectomy could be ill before or after the surgery, careful review by the internist and anesthesia team is required before the decision to proceed to surgery is taken. If the patient is on routine dialysis, heparin-free dialysis may be beneficial in reducing the incidence of intraoperative and postoperative hemorrhage. Preoperative administration of intravitreal VEGF injection has become popular in recent times and has been shown to decrease the rate of intraoperative and postoperative hemorrhage; it also improves intraoperative visibility and reduces surgery time.

Importantly, an internist clearance is required before preoperative adjunctive anti-VEGF is administered to avoid a situation in which following the administration of anti-VEGF, surgery is postponed due to the patient's ill health. This may result in an overactivity of the anti-VEGF with severe contraction of the fibrous component of the fibrovascular membrane resulting in a worsening TRD (and perhaps more retinal ischemia); this is known as a "Crunch." The use of anti-VEGF will be discussed in more detail later on.

4. Preoperative ocular considerations

1. Visual acuity: preoperative acuity has been shown to be an important factor in determining the eventual postoperative visual outcome, with eyes having better preoperative vision tending to have improved postoperative vision. Also, TRD involving the macula will have poorer preoperative vision than a "macular sparing" TRD. Therefore surgery should be performed once the macula is perceived to be threatened. Macular ischemia remains an important reason for poor preoperative and postoperative vision; this can be determined by the use of fundus fluorescein angiography (FFA) to assess for macular non-perfusion. Optical coherence angiography (OCT angiography or OCTA) can also be used and has the advantage of repeatability of the test. However, in several cases, it is not possible to perform this FFA assessment of the macular vasculature before surgery because of opacities in the medium, including VH and FVP, which obscure the view of the macula.

2. Intraocular pressure (IOP): this may be normal or elevated. When IOP is elevated, it is important to assess the anterior chamber angles and anterior uvea carefully, in search of rubeosis. The finding of rubeosis suggests very significant retinal ischemia and further worsens the prognosis for recovery of vision. The rise in IOP may also have damaging effects on the cornea, including cornea edema, and result in decreased visibility during surgery.

3. Cornea: the clarity of this structure is required for proper access and visibility required for diabetic vitrectomy. The use of contact lens viewing systems significantly increases the incidence of cornea opacity and may require the removal of cornea epithelium during the surgery. Such scrapping off of cornea epithelium could result in postoperative cornea defects, which could take some time to heal. The aforementioned situation has been greatly reduced with the more frequent use of non-contact lens viewing systems.

4. Pupil: it is vital to assess for adequate pupillary dilatation prior to surgery. A poorly dilating pupil may require more than pharmacological mydriasis. In some instances pupillary synechiae may exist and will require mechanical dilatation such as using iris hooks.

5. Lens: the presence of significant cataract may require that a combined vitrectomy and cataract removal be performed during the same surgery. The cataract is first removed using a phacoemulsification technique, then the diabetic vitrectomy is performed. The intraocular lens (IOL) could be inserted before or at the conclusion of the vitrectomy. This combined procedure has become a popular technique in recent years. It provides a clearer view and lends itself to improved access to the retina periphery with the use of a wide-angle viewing lens. However, it can also be associated with significant complications of the anterior segment, since there could be enhanced diffusion of the growth factors including VEGF from the posterior segment to the anterior segment of the eye, resulting in the formation of rubeosis iridis and its sequelae.

6. A B scan ultrasound is a useful ocular investigation to have, especially in situations in which there is limited or no view of the retina as a result of vitreous hemorrhage, opacities in the vitreous, and cataract. A B scan can detect the presence or absence of posterior vitreous detachment (PVD) and provide information useful for preparing the eye for diabetic vitrectomy. For instance, some surgeons would give preoperative intravitreal anti-VEGF in eyes without a PVD and refrain from doing so in eyes in which a PVD already exists. Also a B scan can detect the presence of vitreoschisis (aka second membrane). Vitreoschisis is common in diabetic retinopathy eyes, and for this reason re-staining using multiple intravitreal triamcinolone injections is important to detect the residual vitreous layer when vitreoschisis is present. Vitreoschisis is thought to be due to vitreous hemorrhage in the gel splitting the vitreous fibers. Recognizing its presence is essential for good outcome.

5. Relevant pathophysiology and surgical principles

Advanced stages of DR are characterized by retina edema and ischemia, consequent to vascular hyperpermeability and vascular occlusion, respectively. The chronic hyperglycemia results in progressive damage to the retinal capillary network resulting in retinal hypoxia and release of hypoxia-inducible factor (HIF) from the affected areas of the retina. The resultant ischemic retina due to the action of HIF then releases pro angiogenesis growth factors which include basic fibroblast growth factor (FGF), insulinlike growth factor 1 (IGF 1), erythropoietin, and, the most known growth factor, VEGF [29]. Also, cytokines such as IL-6, IL-8, and MCP-1 are released. The interaction of these growth factors and cytokines stimulate angiogenesis. VEGF-mediated new blood vessels sprout out from the surrounding vessels, i.e., capillaries and venules, and invade the vitreous. Progressive vasoproliferation occurs in response to increasing levels of the growth factors; and this is associated with proliferation of fibrous tissue resulting in the characteristic fibrovascular membranes. The fibrovascular tissue proliferates and extends across the retina in the preretinal space (or sub hyaloid space). In eyes with PVD, fibrovascular membranes can only grow on the surface of the retina; therefore, retinal detachments do not tend to occur. However in eyes without a PVD (which is often the case), the posterior hyaloid acts as a scaffold that allows the fibrovascular tissue to grow, leading to traction on the retina and retinal detachments. Tractional forces within the vitreous exert effect on these rather brittle new blood vessels resulting in different degrees of hemorrhage. The resulting hemorrhage can range from a small leakage of blood on the surrounding retina to larger preretinal hemorrhage (**Figure 1a**) and to a more severe break through intragel vitreous hemorrhage.

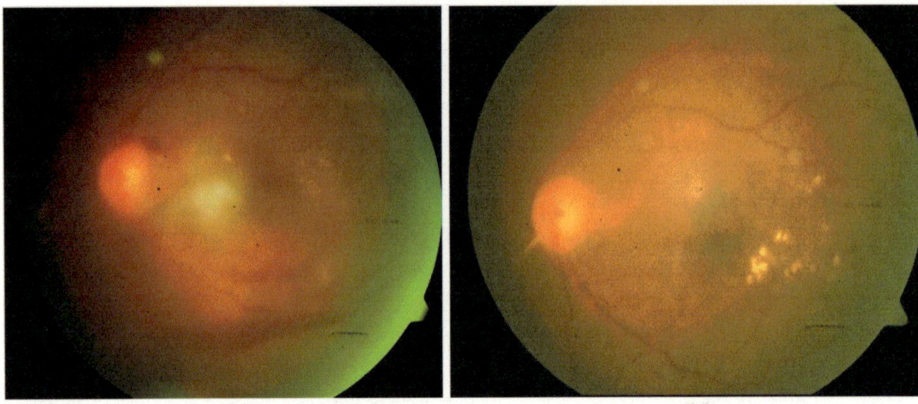

(a) (b)

Figure 1.
Fundus photograph of PDR. (a) Left eye showing diffuse vitreous hemorrhage and preretinal hemorrhage in an eye diagnosed to have PDR. Notice also the absence of retinal laser marks and presence of macula hard exudates, with some significant cataract. (b) Same eye as in 1a after vitrectomy; view of the fundus is clearer and some hard exudates persist in the macular area.

This hemorrhage can often be removed using vitrectomy technique (**Figure 1b**). The fibrous component of the fibrovascular tissue contracts, due to a myofibroblastic effect [30], and causes traction on the inner retina, resulting in a TRD that may initially involve an extra macular site, and then subsequently progresses to the macula and damages vision. In some cases the traction results in a split in the layers of the retina (retinoschisis or foveoschisis) that can be appreciated on optical coherence tomography (OCT) scan. Similarly, ERM may be present in the macular area and result in considerable macular traction, worsening already existing macular edema. Since such diabetic macular edema (DME) has a traction-induced component as its causation, surgery will be required to remove the traction if resolution of the edema is to be achieved. VEGF suppression alone is unlikely to achieve complete resolution of this sort of DME, and this needs to be recognized.

The surgical principles of diabetic vitrectomy include performing a core vitrectomy. In some cases, a posterior vitreous separation already exists preoperatively and the goal of surgery is simply vitreous hemorrhage removal. This is a rather uncommon presentation. In cases of vitreous hemorrhage removal, in addition to the hemorrhage (since the vitreous cavity acts as a reservoir of several pro-inflammatory and pro-angiogenic factors that result in macular edema, neovascularization, and proliferation of fibrous tissue), diabetic vitrectomy also achieves immediate removal of these factors and cytokines. It facilitates access to the retina and permits release of the posterior hyaloid and further dissection of the tractional fibrotic membranes that create the TRD.

Separation of the anterior vitreous from the more posterior cortical vitreous can be easily accomplished using any standard vitreous cutter, allowing the release of the anteroposterior traction induced by the vitreous. Careful dissection of the posterior vitreous cortex from the underlying retina and the removal of proliferating fibrovascular membranes and fibrous bands from the retina surface (and at times from the subretinal space) are the highlights of the surgery. This should be done, avoiding the creation of iatrogenic breaks and creation of false passages. Identification of the right plane of vitreoretinal separation is the key to proper dissection and avoiding unnecessary iatrogenic breaks. One tip to achieve entry into the right vitreoretinal plane in difficult situations is to commence dissection from the optic disc and then move out towards the macula and retina periphery, the "inside out approach." In practice, it is possible to detach the vitreous at the optic disc with gentle traction on the adjoining vitreous or fibrous tissue close to the optic disc using an intraocular forceps or the aspiration port of a vitreous cutter. This lifts the vitreous off the disc and ensures a safe entry into the vitreoretinal space, from where dissection can continue outward. In some cases a moderate to large amount of retrohyaloid blood already exists; this provides a useful entry point into the desired vitreoretinal space.

Techniques for fibrovascular proliferation removal have been well described and include en bloc dissection in which vitreous and proliferating tissue is removed as one, segmentation of fibrovascular tissue into islands of tissue using straight scissors or small-gauge cutter, and delamination involving careful removal of the islands of tissue using a small-gauge cutter or a curved intraocular scissors [31, 32]. Various ancillary instrumentation including picks, vertical and horizontal scissors, blades, membrane peeler cutters, forceps, scrapers, and other instruments can be used for the removal of proliferating fibrovascular membranes. However the use of newer high cut rate multifunctional vitreous cutters enables surgeons to often complete TRD repair using only the vitreous cutter [33, 34].

Upon completion of membrane dissection, ERM in the macular area may require identification and removal. Subretinal fluid drainage may be required. Existing retinal ischemia is treated with the application of laser panretinal photocoagulation [35]. PRP should be done up to the extreme retinal periphery, i.e., ora serrata. Scleral indentation is performed in search of iatrogenic retina breaks (which if undetected and treated can result in postoperative RRD and need for re-vitrectomy). Indentation is also done to ensure PRP has been extended to all areas of peripheral ischemia. Some surgeon will apply cryotherapy to the peripheral retina, to ensure maximum obliteration of the ischemic drive.

There may be a need for longer acting tamponade such as silicone oil in the more complex retina detachments such as in TRD cases with the occurrence of significant iatrogenic breaks, TRD/RRD situation, or in cases with existing traction [36]. Silicone oil is also used in monocular patients and patients who cannot position or who have to undertake air travel soon. Otherwise air, saline or shorter acting tamponade such as SF6 is sufficient in cases of low to medium complexity, especially if there are no iatrogenic breaks and release of traction is considered adequate. C3F8 can be used if longer duration of tamponade is required. It is important to ensure that sclerotomy ports are well closed, with no leakage. If required and judged to be necessary, sclerotomy sites should be sutured using, e.g., 8-0 vicryl suture, to prevent hypotony and reduce the risk of postoperative vitreous hemorrhage. A reported disadvantage of the sutured sclerotomy is postoperative patient discomfort and induction of cornea astigmatism, which tends to settle and return to preoperative status over some weeks.

6. Intraoperative considerations

Diabetic vitrectomy has benefited from the overwhelming advances that have occurred in vitrectomy over the past decade. This includes advances in surgical technique, instrumentation, improved preoperative patient work-up, and case selection. All this has resulted in improved surgical outcome, which has further increased surgeon confidence in performing surgery, even in the more complex vitreoretinal cases. Some of these advances in diabetic vitrectomy and their impact are as enumerated and discussed below:

1. Improvements in vitrectomy machines and probes, which includes faster cutting rates and smaller gauges (27 G, 25 G, and 23 G) trans conjunctival vitrectomy

systems, now means that these probes can be used as multifunctional tools. They can be inserted carefully beneath tractional membranes during surgery and used effectively for segmentation and delamination of the membranes without the need for intraocular scissors in several cases. Also the high cut rates provide for less traction on the retina, reduce the mobility of the retina, and reduce the rate of iatrogenic breaks. The presence of the vitrectomy cutting port closer to the tip of the probes means that membranes on the retina can be easily engaged. Indeed many complex cases can be safely completed with the use of only the vitreous cutter and no other ancillary instruments required. Similarly the protection conferred by the cannula system at the sclerotomy entry site provides for reduced incidence of entry sight breaks, vitreous incarceration at the wound edge, and leaking sclerotomies.

2. The introduction of intraoperative self-retaining lighting systems, such as the chandelier illuminating system, provides a free hand which can be used to grasp and stabilize intraocular tissue with a forceps while a fibrovascular membrane (FVM) is being dissected away. This led to the use of bimanual surgical technique. Bimanual surgery provides a very useful means of membrane dissection in difficult TRD and TRD/RRD cases, with broad attachment of fibrovascular membrane to the retina. Also various illuminated instruments, such as the lighted peaks, can provide considerable support in membrane dissection and relief of traction.

3. During the early days of diabetic vitrectomy, as the era of the DRVS, the ability to perform endoretinal photocoagulation was lacking. The presence of endoretinal photocoagulation probes has provided additional stabilization to the surgery outcome, since panretinal laser photocoagulation can now be done during the surgery irrespective of the occurrence of postoperative vitreous cavity hemorrhage. Supplemental retinal laser photocoagulation may be required in addition to already existing retinal laser marks. PRP should be adequate and done up to the retina periphery to cover the ischemic retina and prevent postoperative complications such as recurrent hemorrhage or AHFVP.

4. The intraoperative use of triamcinolone crystals to highlight the posterior vitreous cortex has helped visualization and improves complete removal of the vitreous. In some cases vitreoschisis is present, and this can be detected if the additional triamcinolone is used. Also vital dyes such as brilliant blue G (BBG) and membrane blue (MB) have been found to help in highlighting ERM and ILM, therefore facilitating its removal. While the removal of ILM is justified in the macula to prevent re-proliferation of membranes, in some cases this can be quiet difficult, especially in the presence of significant macular edema, with pathologically adherent ILM. In such cases with a risk of further trauma to the macula, ILM peel is best avoided. Injection of PFCL, which acts to stabilize the retina during the ILM peel, in some cases, may improve the chances of successful ILM peel.

5. Obtaining a preoperative OCT has become a standard work-up procedure for eyes with diabetic retinopathy (**Figure 2a**). Aside from providing useful histological overview of the retina and vitreous, it can be used to provide three-dimensional overlay including showing areas of vitreoretinal adhesion, pegs as they are called, and areas of vitreous separation, which is important for surgical planning. Also it provides additional information on prognosis for postoperative vision, since eyes with more preoperative preserved external

DOI: http://dx.doi.org/10.5772/intechopen.91360

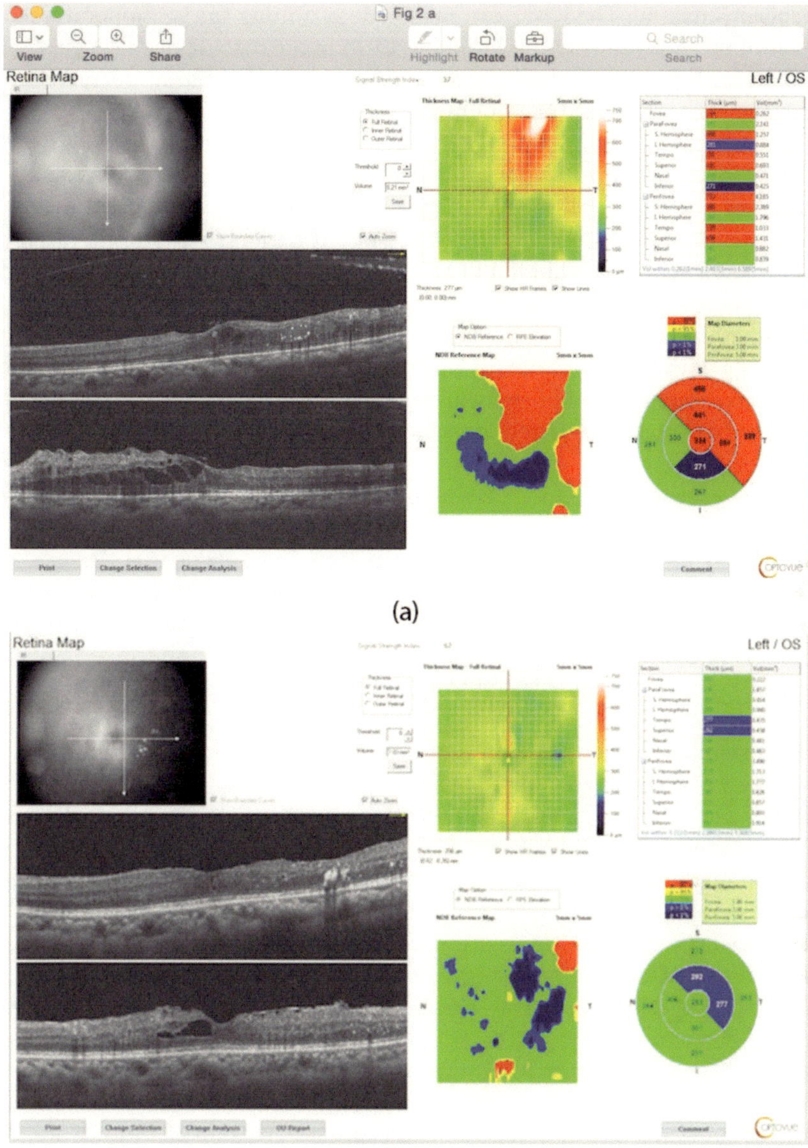

Figure 2.
OCT images of same patient whose fundus picture is shown above. (a) Preoperative crossline OCT images of the same eye as in ***Figure 1a****. Notice the presence of localized macular edema and vitreous hemorrhage with PVD. (b) Postoperative OCT images with normal subfoveal thickness but some intraretinal cystic spaces.*

limiting membrane (ELM) and ellipsoid zone (EZ) layers (as in **Figure 2a**) have been demonstrated to have better postoperative vision than eyes without, since a preserved EZ and ELM are also expected after surgery (**Figure 2b**). The postoperative presence of EZ and ELM, which are outer retinal layers, are essential predictors of postoperative recovery of vision.

Fairly decent OCT images can be obtained in eyes with a limited amount of vitreous hemorrhage as in **Figure 2a**. Unfortunately in some of the eyes with an obscured view of the retina, OCT is not possible. However, the successful incorporation of OCT technology into the operating microscope provides the intraoperative OCT (iOCT), which has shown usefulness in intraoperative decision-making. The iOCT can help in determining the intraoperative presence of unremoved traction inducing ERM in the macula or the occurrence of a macular hole, which requires to be addressed during the surgery, since this can significantly affect postoperative visual outcome.

6. Timing of surgery: there is considerable interest in improving the visual outcome of eyes undergoing diabetic vitrectomy. This has resulted in some advocacy for earlier surgery in the category of patients with proliferative disease, instead of waiting for progression to more advanced TRD. Also efforts at inducing a pharmacologic separation of the vitreous from the retina using enzymatic vitreolysis have not been rewarding. Much of diabetic vitrectomy has to do with the separation of the attached vitreous. Induction of posterior vitreous separation could significantly halt the progression of PDR, since the attached vitreous is required for continued FVP.

On the other hand, there are advocates for caution in diabetic vitrectomy, who argue for the more aggressive use of a combination of intravitreal anti-VEGF and retinal laser photocoagulation. They argue that the outcome of diabetic vitrectomy could be unpredictable and that even in seemingly straightforward cases, intra- and postoperative complications was not uncommon. Diabetic vitrectomy according to them should be undertaken only when necessary and other medical options exhausted.

7. Pharmacologic adjuvants: In recent times the use of pharmacological therapy has been introduced as adjuvant for use preoperatively and intraoperatively in diabetic vitrectomy. Intravitreal Injection of anti-VEGFs including Macugen, Avastin, and Lucentis has been used preoperatively and postoperatively, while steroid implants such as Ozurdex have been used pre- and intraoperatively.

Bevacizumab (Avastin, Genentech, South San Francisco, CA, USA) appears to be the most commonly used preoperative anti-VEGF injection [37, 38]. Preoperative injection of anti-VEGF agents is known to considerably shrink neovascular fronds and has been shown to reduce intraoperative and postoperative bleeding and result in improved visual outcome [38–42]. However, an overaction of anti-VEGF can cause contraction of fibrovascular membrane and could exacerbate the traction and cause progression of TRD, in some cases causing a macular sparing TRD to involve the macula. This has been called the "crunch syndrome" which is characterized by a worsening tractional retinal detachment and development of denser fibrotic connections between the retina and overlying tissue, which makes it harder to identify tissue planes and results in more difficult dissection of the fibrous membranes [43].

Therefore the optimum time for anti-VEGF injection preoperatively should be enough time to cause the desired effect, which is reduction in neovascularization, and not long enough to induce severe fibrotic contraction and worsening of TRD. It is generally thought that the ideal time frame is somewhere between 3 and 5 days prior to surgery, with considerable variation among surgeons. This time frame enables neovascular regression while limiting fibrovascular membrane contraction.

Pegaptanib (Macugen, Bausch, and Lomb, Bridgewater, NJ, USA) has been used as an adjunct, when injected preoperatively. Pegaptanib is a PEGylated aptamer and only inhibits the VEGF isoform 165 [44]. It therefore has been suggested to have a more selective effect on the neovascularization component of the fibrovascular membrane and less tractional effect with lower systemic risks [44].

Therefore it can be used to induce regression of neovascularization, in a way similar to bevacizumab, and therefore reduces the risk of intraoperative bleeding, but does not have a similar tractional effect as seen with the use of bevacizumab [45]. This may allow for injection of Pegaptanib at any given time prior to surgery, even in the form of multiple injections, awaiting physician clearance, and good timing for surgery. There is however no wide spread use of Pegaptanib for this purpose, and comparison with bevacizumab has not been done. It may also be systemically advantageous due to the lower risk of vascular accidents in these high-risk patients [44]. It is instructive to mention that Pegaptanib is rarely used as an anti-VEGF of choice for suppression of VEGF in other neovascular ocular pathologies.

Ozurdex (Allergan, Dublin, Ireland) is a biodegradable 0.7 mg dexamethasone implant that is injected intravitreally via a 22-gauge needle and has been approved by the Food and Drug Administration (FDA) for the treatment of DME. It has been used in the pre- and postoperative control of the neovascularization process and tissue edema. As noted by Mahmoud et al., it can be injected preoperatively in an eye with extensive TRD in which it facilitates regression and consolidation of neovascularization in addition to inhibiting other inflammatory cytokines [45]. Unlike anti-VEGF agents, it is not known to increase risk of systemic complications, and there is no associated fibrovascular membrane or retinal tractional response. Tissue planes were found to be more distinct and not changed into flat fibrovascular tissue, making them more difficult to dissect, as was seen following administration of anti-VEGF agents. Due to these properties, it provides for flexibility with operative physician clearance planning (there is adequate time for preoperative clearance when Ozurdex is being used). In addition, the effect of Ozurdex can continue well into the postoperative period, since the Ozurdex implant can remain in position in the postoperative period under silicone oil [45]. Ozurdex implant releases the active drug over a period of 6 months and therefore keeps the eyes quiet, and the neovascular process is inactive during the postoperative period.

8. Techniques and tips for fibrovascular membrane dissection. Certain techniques are useful in the safe removal of fibrovascular tissue. The following are by no means exhaustive and are at best suggestions:

    a. Smaller-gauge (25 G and 27 G) transconjunctival surgery can provide opportunity for the vitrectomy probe to be inserted between the membrane and the retina. Using an aspiration mode, the membrane is lifted up with the cutting edge of the probe facing superiorly. As soon as resistance to the membrane lifting is encountered, the membrane is cut with the cutter. In this way the fibrovascular membrane is segmented; then the islands of fibrovascular tissue are removed from the retina using a delamination technique. Using the probe in this fashion, it can also serve as a blunt dissector and can be used without the need for additional instrumentation such as scissors or pick.

    b. Viscodissection is a very useful technique in cases of very adherent membranes [46, 47]. It was born from the idea that the use of liquid or fluid instead of metal or other materials to separate membranes from normal retina would have safety advantages. The use of small tip retractable cannulas, which can be inserted into small spaces between fibrovascular membranes and detached or attached retina, enables injection of hyaluronic acid (HA). The HA serves to separate the membrane from the retina, and the viscodissection cannula can be used for blunt dissection as well. In addition, the HA provides hemostasis and improves visibility in the area of the dissection. Care should be taken to ensure adequate removal of the HA after the surgery to prevent a rise in IOP.

c. In the extremely difficult cases of TRD and TRD/RRD, characterized by thickened fibrotic membranes strongly adherent to the retina, a combination of forceps with curved scissors is a good option. With the use of a bimanual technique using a chandelier illumination placed at 12 O clock position (or any other position as chosen by the surgeon) and wide-angle viewing, the edge of thickened fibrovascular membranes can be engaged using a good gripping tissue forceps and then separated from the retina with scissors. After the separation, the membrane or clot can then be cut off with the small-gauge cutter using reduced cut rates.

d. Proportional reflux is a feature of the Constellation vitrectomy machine and other machines that have been used in the safe dissection of membranes from the normal retina [48]. The Constellation Vision System (Alcon Laboratories, Fort Worth, TX) has the pulse reflux mode, which allows a jet of fluid to be ejected from the port and is useful for ejecting accidentally incarcerated tissue during vitrectomy. In addition to this, it also has a proportional reflux mode. The proportional reflux mode allows for fluid to be ejected from the vitrectomy probe port in a gradual and controlled manner with foot pedal control, thus the term proportional reflux. The concurrent development of microincisional vitrectomy surgery with a smaller gauge and the port being closer to the tip as well as the development of proportional reflux has allowed for a new surgical technique known as "proportional reflux hydrodissection" [48, 49]. In this technique, credited to Dugel, the port of the cutter is placed between the fibrovascular tissue and the normal retinal tissue. Thereafter, with the foot pedal, the surgeon has complete control over fluid extrusion in a proportional fashion to create a separation between the fibrous tissue and the normal retina.

7. Complications of surgery

Vitrectomy in an eye that suffers from PDR can have significant complications. This ought to be considered and the risk for these intra- and postoperative complication considered before the decision to perform surgery is taken. Some of these complications include intra- and postoperative vitreous cavity hemorrhage (early or delayed), recurrent vitreous hemorrhage, hypotony, progression of diabetic retinopathy, iatrogenic retinal breaks (commonly occurring during fibrovascular tissue dissection), cornea edema, sclerotomy-related complications including vitreous incarceration (not as common with small-gauge vitrectomy compared to 20 G era), vascular ingrowths and AHFVP, rapid progression of cataract, phototoxicity (associated with chandelier illumination placement close to the retina), rubeosis and rubeotic glaucoma (more common in pseudophakia and aphakia), and severe loss of vision. Rubeotic glaucoma is a troublesome disease to manage and will require the use of intravitreal anti-VEGF, retinal laser photocoagulation, or cryotherapy. In some cases additional cyclodestructive procedure or glaucoma drainage tube surgery may be indicated. Fortunately the incidence of this complication is on the decline due to the use of laser endo photocoagulation, which enables more aggressive management of the peripheral ischemia.

Much of the complications can be avoided with meticulous attention to currently available surgical techniques. For instance, the rate of intra- and postoperative hemorrhage can be reduced by the use of preoperative intravitreal anti-VEGF as previously described and careful hemostasis during surgery either by the elevation of intraocular pressure, cautious diathermy, direct application of pressure to bleeding vessels, or application of viscoelastic to the point of bleeding. Also preoperative discontinuation of blood thinners and attention to the systemic blood pressure during and after surgery to ensure it is not elevated can be helpful.

8. Outcome

In recent times due to improvements witnessed in vitrectomy technology and technique as previously discussed, the anatomical and visual outcome of diabetic vitrectomy has generally improved. Compared to the earlier era, when endoretinal laser photocoagulation for treating retinal ischemia intraoperatively was not available (retinal ischemia is the main drive for the proliferative retinal changes), we now have a host of retinal laser photocoagulation probes available for use during vitrectomy. There have been reports of improvements in visual acuity in 75% and 87% of TRD eyes and vitreous hemorrhage eyes, respectively [50, 51]. With continued improvements and probably earlier timing of surgery, success rates will likely continue to improve and may exceed the 90% rates. Some of the poor prognostic factors include poor pre-op visual acuity, rubeosis, ectopia or displacement, and macula involving TRD. Significant fovea ischemia, which can be recognized with the use of fundus fluorescein angiography and OCTA, has a poor prognosis.

To conclude, diabetic vitrectomy has benefited from the advances in the sphere of vitreoretinal surgery. Though presentation of proliferative DR is very variable and can be complex, modern tools and technique can in most cases improve or stabilize vision. There is an ongoing discussion on possible identification of eyes at risk for progression and offering earlier surgery. This may result in further improvements. Perhaps the development of an ideal pharmacologic vitreolytic agent which will induce a PVD in eyes known to have PDR will usher in a new era in diabetic vitrectomy.

Acknowledgements

I wish to expresses my thanks to Dr Vipin Vig, vitreoretinal surgeon in Amritsar, India, who took the time to read through my manuscript and made useful suggestions.

Conflict of interest

None.

Author details

Ogugua N. Okonkwo
Eye Foundation Retina Institute, Lagos, Nigeria

*Address all correspondence to: o_okonkwo@yahoo.com

References

[1] Ogurtsova K, da Rocha Fernandes JD, Huang Y, et al. IDF Diabetes Atlas: Global estimates for the prevalence of diabetes for 2015 and 2040. Diabetes Research and Clinical Practice. 2017;**128**:40-50

[2] Yau JW, Rogers SL, Kawasaki R, et al. Global prevalence and major risk factors of diabetic retinopathy. Diabetes Care. 2012;**35**:556-564

[3] Leasher JL, Bourne RR, Flaxman SR, et al. Global estimates on the number of people blind or visually impaired by diabetic retinopathy: A meta-analysis from 1990 to 2010. Diabetes Care. 2016;**39**:1643-1649

[4] Sabanayagam C, Banu R, Chee ML, et al. Incidence and progression of diabetic retinopathy: A systematic review. The Lancet Diabetes & Endocrinology. Feb 2019;7(2):140-149. DOI: 10.1016/s2213-8587(18)30128-1

[5] Wirkkala J, Bloigu R, Hautala NM. Intravitreal bevacizumab improves the clearance of vitreous haemorrhage and visual outcomes in patients with proliferative diabetic retinopathy. BMJ Open Ophthalmology. 2019;**4**(1):e000390. DOI: 10.1136/bmjophth-2019-000390

[6] Zhou AY, Zhou CJ, Yao J, Quan YL, Ren BC, Wang JM. Panretinal photocoagulation versus panretinal photocoagulation plus intravitreal bevacizumab for high-risk proliferative diabetic retinopathy. International Journal of Ophthalmology. 2016;**9**(12):1772-1778. DOI: 10.18240/ijo.2016.12.12

[7] Someya H, Takayama K, Takeuchi M, et al. Outcomes of 25-gauge vitrectomy for tractional and nontractional diabetic macular edema with proliferative diabetic retinopathy. Journal of Ophthalmology. 2019;**2019**:5304524. DOI: 10.1155/2019/5304524

[8] Newman DK. Surgical management of the late complications of proliferative diabetic retinopathy. Eye (London). 2010;**24**(3):441-449

[9] Qamar RM, Saleem MI, Saleem MF. The outcomes of pars plana vitrectomy without endotamponade for tractional retinal detachment secondary to proliferative diabetic retinopathy. International Journal of Ophthalmology. 2013;**6**(5):671-674. DOI: 10.3980/j.issn.2222-3959.2013.05.23

[10] Shen YD, Yang CM. Extended silicone oil tamponade in primary vitrectomy for complex retinal detachment in proliferative diabetic retinopathy: A long-term follow-up study. European Journal of Ophthalmology. 2007;**17**(6):954-960

[11] Fujii GY, De Juan E Jr, Humayun MS, et al. A new 25-gauge instrument system for transconjunctival sutureless vitrectomy surgery. Ophthalmology. 2002;**109**(10):1807-1812

[12] Eckardt C. Transconjunctival sutureless 23-gauge vitrectomy. Retina. 2005;**25**(2):208-211

[13] Oshima Y, Wakabayashi T, Sato T, Ohji M, Tano Y. A 27-gauge instrument system for transconjunctival sutureless microincision vitrectomy surgery. Ophthalmology. 2010;**117**(1):93-102.e2. DOI: 10.1016/j.ophtha.2009.06.043

[14] Abulon DJ, Buboltz DC. Performance comparison of high-speed dual-pneumatic vitrectomy cutters during simulated vitrectomy with balanced salt solution. Translational Vision Science & Technology. 2015;**4**(1):6

[15] Machemer R. Reminiscences after 25 years of pars plana vitrectomy. American Journal of Ophthalmology. 1995;**119**(4):505-510. DOI: 10.1016/s0002-9394(14)71238-3

[16] The Diabetic Retinopathy Vitrectomy Study Research Group. Early vitrectomy for severe vitreous hemorrhage in diabetic retinopathy. Four-year results of a randomized trial: Diabetic Retinopathy Vitrectomy Study Report 5. Archives of Ophthalmology. 1990;**108**:958-964

[17] Diabetic Retinopathy Clinical Research Network Writing Committee, Haller JA, Qin H, Apte RS, et al. Vitrectomy outcomes in eyes with diabetic macular edema and vitreomacular traction. Ophthalmology. 2010;**117**:1087-1093

[18] Stewart MW, Browning DJ, Landers MB. Current management of diabetic tractional retinal detachments. Indian Journal of Ophthalmology. 2018;**66**(12):1751-1762. DOI: 10.4103/ijo.IJO_1217_18

[19] Yau GL, Silva PS, Arrigg PG, Sun JK. Postoperative complications of pars plana vitrectomy for diabetic retinal disease. Seminars in Ophthalmology. 2018;**33**(1):126-133. DOI: 10.1080/08820538.2017.1353832

[20] Berrocal MH, Acaba LA, Acaba A. Surgery for diabetic eye complications. Current Diabetes Reports. 2016;**16**(10):99. DOI: 10.1007/s11892-016-0787-6

[21] Vaziri K, Schwartz SG, Relhan N, Kishor KS, Flynn HW Jr. New therapeutic approaches in diabetic retinopathy. The Review of Diabetic Studies. 2015;**12**:196-210

[22] Cruz-Iñigo YJ, Acabá LA, Berrocal MH. Surgical management of retinal diseases: PROLIFERATIVE diabetic retinopathy and traction retinal detachment. Developments in Ophthalmology. 2014;**54**:196-203. DOI: 10.1159/000360467

[23] Okonkwo ON, Lewis K, Hassan AO, Gyasi ME, Oluyadi B, et al. Indications and outcomes of vitrectomy surgery in a series of 1000 black African eyes. BMJ Open Ophthalmology. 2019;**4**(1):e000083. DOI: 10.1136/bmjophth-2017-000083

[24] Law JC, Sharma AG, Eliott D. Indications for diabetic vitrectomy in African Americans versus Caucasians. Investigative Ophthalmology & Visual Science. 2006;**47**:3835

[25] Aylward B, Tadayoni R, Arevalo F, Karkhaneh R. Anterior hyaloid fibrovascular proliferation. Journal of Ophthalmic & Vision Research. 2010;**5**(1):61-64

[26] Hassan AO, Okonkwo ON, Oderinlo O, Oluyadi F, Ogunro A, Harriman A, et al. Anterior hyaloidal fibrovascular proliferation (AHFVP) in a diabetic after cataract extraction, resulting in hyphaema and vitreous haemorrhage during YAG laser capsulotomy. Nigerian Journal of Ophthalmology. 2009;**17**(1):23-26

[27] Helbig H, Kellner U, Bornfeld N, Foerster MH. Life expectancy of diabetic patients undergoing vitreous surgery. The British Journal of Ophthalmology. 1996;**80**:640-643

[28] Nguyen-Khoa BA, Goehring EL, Werther W, et al. Hospitalized cardiovascular events in patients with diabetic macular edema. BMC Ophthalmology. 2012;**12**:11. DOI: 10.1186/1471-2415-12-11

[29] Abcouwer SF. Angiogenic factors and cytokines in diabetic retinopathy. Journal of Clinical and Cellular Immunology. 2013;Suppl 1(11):1-12

[30] Tamaki K, Usui-Ouchi A, Murakami A, Ebihara N. Fibrocytes and fibrovascular membrane formation in proliferative diabetic retinopathy. Investigative Ophthalmology & Visual Science. 2016;**57**:4999-5005

[31] Gafencu O. Surgical principles and techniques in severe proliferative diabetic retinopathy. Oftalmologia. 2001;**52**:54-57

[32] Miller SA, Butler JB, Myers FL, Bresnick GH. Pars plana vitrectomy. Treatment for tractional macula detachment secondary to proliferative diabetic retinopathy. Archives of Ophthalmology. 1980;**98**:659-664

[33] Celik E, Sever O, Horozoglu F, Yanyalı A. Segmentation and removal of fibrovascular membranes with high-speed 23 G transconjunctival sutureless vitrectomy, in severe proliferative diabetic retinopathy. Clinical Ophthalmology. 2016;**10**:903-910. DOI: 10.2147/OPTH.S95145

[34] Rizzo S, Ebert-Genovesi F, Belting C. Comparative study between a standard 25-gauge vitrectomy system and a new ultrahigh-speed 25-gauge system with duty cycle control in the treatment of various vitreoretinal diseases. Retina. 2011;**31**(10):2007-2013

[35] Gupta V, Arevalo JF. Surgical management of diabetic retinopathy. Middle East African Journal of Ophthalmology. 2013;**20**(4):283-292. DOI: 10.4103/0974-9233.120003

[36] Falkner C, Binder S, Kruger A. Outcome after silicone oil removal. The British Journal of Ophthalmology. 2001;**85**:1324-1327

[37] Avery RL, Pearlman J, Pieramici DJ, et al. Intravitreal bevacizumab (Avastin) in the treatment of proliferative diabetic retinopathy. Ophthalmology. 1695;**2006**(113):e1-e15

[38] Rizzo S, Genovesi-Ebert F, Di Bartolo E, Vento A, Miniaci S, Williams G. Injection of intravitreal bevacizumab (Avastin) as a preoperative adjunct before vitrectomy surgery in the treatment of severe proliferative retinopathy (PDR). Graefe Archive for Clinical and Experimental Ophthalmology. 2008;**246**:837-842

[39] da R Lucena D, Ribeiro JA, Costa RA, Barbosa JC, Scott IU, de Figueiredo-PontesLL,etal.Intraoperative bleeding during vitrectomy for diabetic tractional detachment with versus without preoperative intravitreal bevacizumab. British Journal of Ophthalmology. 2009;**93**:688-691

[40] Modarres M, Nazari H, Falavarjani KG, Naseripour M, Hashemi M, Parvaresh MM. Intravitreal injection of bevacizumab before vitrectomy for proliferative diabetic retinopathy. European Journal of Ophthalmology. 2009;**19**:848-852

[41] Gupta A, Bansal R, Gupta V, Dogra MR. Six-month visual outcome after pars plana vitrectomy in proliferative diabetic retinopathy with or without a single postoperative injection of intravitreal bevacizumab. International Ophthalmology. 2012;**32**:135-144

[42] Ushida H, Kachi S, Asami T, Ishikawa K, Kondo M, Terasaki H. Influence of preoperative intravitreal bevacizumab on visual function in eyes with proliferative diabetic retinopathy. Ophthalmic Research. 2013;**49**:30-36

[43] Arevalo JF, Maia M, Flynn HW Jr, Saravia M, Avery RL, Wu L, et al. Tractional retinal detachment following intravitreal bevacizumab (Avastin) in patients with severe proliferative diabetic retinopathy. The British Journal of Ophthalmology. 2008;**92**:213-216

[44] Nagpal M, Nagpal K, Nagpal PN. A comparative debate on the various anti-vascular endothelial growth factor drugs: Pegaptanib sodium (Macugen), ranibizumab (Lucentis) and

bevacizumab (Avastin). Indian Journal of Ophthalmology. 2007;**55**:437-439

[45] Oellers P, Mahmoud TH. Surgery for proliferative diabetic retinopathy: New tips and tricks. Journal of Ophthalmic & Vision Research. 2016;**11**(1):93-99. DOI: 10.4103/2008-322X.180697

[46] Crafoord S, Stenkula S. Healon GV in posterior segment surgery. Acta Ophthalmologica. 1993;**71**:560-561

[47] Stenkula S, Ivert L, Berglin L, Crafoord S. Healon Yellow as a surgical tool in maneuvering intraocular tissues. Ophthalmic Surgery. 1992;**23**:708-710

[48] Dugel PU. Proportional reflux hydrodissection. Retina. 2012;**32**(3):629-630. DOI: 10.1097/iae.0b013e31824453c7

[49] Jain S, Agarwal A, Aggarwal K, Gupta V. The role of proportional reflux during pars plana vitrectomy for tractional retinal detachments. Ophthalmic Surgery, Lasers and Imaging Retina. 2019;**50**(2):113-115. DOI: 10.3928/23258160-20190129-08

[50] Tao Y, Jiang YR, Li XX, Gao L, Jonas JB. Long-term results of vitrectomy without endotamponade in proliferative diabetic retinopathy with tractional retinal detachment. Retina. 2010;**30**:447-451

[51] Gupta B, Sivaprasad S, Wong R, et al. Visual and anatomical outcomes following vitrectomy for complications of diabetic retinopathy: The DRIVE UK study. Eye (London, England). 2012;**26**:510-516

Section 2

The Foot in Diabetes

Chapter 4

Introductory Chapter: Diabetic Foot

Meriem Braiki, Mohamed Ali Khalifa, Bilel Faidi, Mosaab Ghannouchi and Fethi Derbel

1. Introduction

Diabetic foot disease is an important problem confronting the diabetologist, internists, and surgeons as it reduces patient's quality of life and affects social participation. It is including several chronic complications as infection, foot ulceration and even tissue destruction of the foot. These complications are considered as a significant cause of morbidity and mortality among diabetic patients. Consequently, chronic complications or diabetic foot disease are a growing concern worldwide and represent a major global medical, social, and economic problem.

Diabetic Foot Ulcer (DFU) is one of the most distressing complications and it is defined as the commonest major end-point of diabetic foot disease.

The main etiological factors for DFU are peripheral nerves damage and peripheral vascular disease. Series of mechanisms are documented such as decreased peripheral blood flow and decreased local angiogenesis.

Furthermore, biomechanical abnormalities and increased susceptibility for infection are associated factors exposing to DFU [1, 2].

2. Etiopathogenesis

The etipathogenesis of diabetic foot disease is multifactorial with major factors. Neuropathy, microvascular disease and infection are mainly included. These factors are leading to foot tissue necrosis and ulcer occurrence [2, 3].

2.1 Neuropathy in diabetic foot

About 50% of patients with diabetes mellitus develop symptomatic peripheral neuropathy within 25 years of disease onset. Distal polyneuropathy is commonly encountered. Whereas combined neuropathies with motor and autonomic fibers involvement can occur. Age, disease duration and poor glyceamic control quality over several years are strong predictors, leading to diabetic neuropathy [4].

Hyperglycemia, dyslipidemia, insulin resistance and oxidative stress can contribute to diabetic neuropathy [5].

According to Rochester Study [6], the severity of the neuropathy is related to the duration of hyperglycemia exposure. Other factors are studied in current researchs focusing on oxidative stress, advanced glycation-end products, protein kinase C and the polyol pathway [7].

IntechOpen

2.2 Vasculopathy

Peripheral vascular disease is among the main etiological factors in foot ulceration. Chronic hyperglycemia causes peripheral arteries damage, smooth cell abnormalities and endothelial cell dysfunction.

Endothelial dysfunction, owing to changes in the proliferation of endothelial cells, thickening of the basement membrane, leads essentially to microvascular disease which is responsible for ischemia. Hyperglycemia is also associated with an increase in thromboxane A2 leading to plasma hypercoagulability [8].

2.3 Immunopathy

The immune system is compromised with hyperglycemia and research indicates the impairment of the immune system with serum glucose levels exceeding to 150 ml/dl. Thus, high blood glucose levels lead to inappropriate inflammatory response and disruption of cellular immunity (inhibition of fibroblast proliferation and impairment of the basal layer of keratinocytes, reducing epidermal cell migration) [8].

Consequently, diabetic patients are more exosed to the foot infection which is a limb-threatening and debilitating condition mainly seen in incontrolled diabetes. The soft tissue infection adversely affects diabetic control. This repetitive cycle leads to uncontrolled hyperglycemia, further affecting the immune response to infection [9]. The bone can be involved in case of infection resistance responsible for soft tissue infection dissemination making osteitis.

Bad glycemia control associated with an open wound creates a catabolic state and a metabolic dysfunction affecting the synthesis of proteins, collagen and fibroblasts. Furthermore, systemic deficiencies are propagated leading to nutritional compromise in diabetes [10].

3. Classification

Many classifications of the diabetic foot are reported. The most commonly used is Wagner's classification, consisting of six simplistic wound grades used to assess ulcer depth (grades 0–5) [11]. This classification is limited as it is not able to recognize ischaemia and infection as independent risk factors in all classification grades [12]. A more recently proposed and popularized DFU classification is the University of Texas Wound Classification [13].

4. Clinical presentation

Clinical foot examination at each follow-up is important to detect the disease early such as ulceration or gangrene. The clinical examination includes inspection of the skin integrity, foot deformities such as, Charcot's foot, hallux valgus, claw toe, hollow foot, skew or flat foot. The muscular condition and the bone structure should be evaluated as well [4].

Hyperkeratosis with dry and fissured skin are features of polyneuropathy. Lower extremity vascular insufficiency is made by one or more signs of claudication, night or rest pain, atrophic integument, absent peripheral pulses and loss of limb hair [8].

About 50% of patients with DFU present clinical signs of infection which is clinically featured by the presence of purulent secretions or at least two of the inflammatory classic signs (painful swelling, edema, hyperemia). The lack of the sensitivity in patients with impaired immune response due to neuropathy can make these signs masked [8].

5. Investigations

Guideline development group selected recommendations from the National Institute of Clinical Excellence. In their most recent publishment, the annual assessment of the diabetic foot requires recommendations aiming essentially to assess both of peripheral neuropathy and peripheral vascular status.

Peripheral vascular disease is diagnosed by angiography which studies the peripheral arterial tree. Non-invasive vascular screening is currently more used in the diabetic foot to detect early the peripheral ischemia [14].

These investigations consist of Doppler ultrasound (for estimation of ankle brachial ratio), photo-plethysmography, transcutaneous oximetry, laser Doppler flowmetry and television microscopy [2].

Most guidelines recommend the use of Neurological foot testing with 10 g monofilament in order to assess diabetic neuropathy. An inability to sense a 10 g pressure is the current consensus definition of loss of protective sensation [15].

6. Management

The management of the diabetic foot complications is multidisciplinary and requires the collaboration of a specialist team comprising a dialectologist, surgeons, podiatrist, microbiologist, tissue viability nurse with a thorough understanding of foot function.

The aim is to decrease the risk of the disease progression leading to feet deformities, ulcers and foot amputation. The prognosis is mainly highlighted by factors such as glycaemic and blood pressure control, diabetic nephropathy and diabetic retinopathy [16].

6.1 Conservative therapeutic modalities

6.1.1 Glycemic control

It is demonstrating that a good controlled glycaemia delays the onset and slows the progression of diabetic neuropathy, retinopathy and nephropathy in patients with insulin-dependent diabetes mellitus [17, 18].

Callaghan et al. [12] showed the decrease in the risk of developing clinical neuropathy with better glycaemic control, in diabetes requiring insulinotherapy.

6.1.2 Pharmacological therapy

The medication adherence to oral diabetic drugs is improved by the patient education. The pain resulting from the distal neuropathy requires the use of pain killers. The National Institute of Clinical Excellence recommends use of first-line agent duloxetine and pregabalin for pain control [19].

Various risk factors for atherosclerosis mainly smoking, should be completely stopped in diabetic patients in order to decrease the risk of distal vascular disease. Adding to that the use of statins and antiplatelet medications reduce the limb ischemia risk and the vascularisation, when it is improved, it is in turn associated with a reduced amputation rate.

A targeted antibiotherapy based on the wound culture results is needed in DFU with superadded infection. The duration of treatment depends on the underlying infection severity [20].

6.1.3 Debridement

A 10-year review on standardized wound care protocol and integrated multidisciplinary team showed a reduction in amputation rate in diabetic foot patients as they had not delayed debridement [21].

Disease activity is measured by the degree of swelling, erythema and especially skin temperature. Superficial ulcer requires the removal of necrotic and hyperkeratotic tissue as it promotes better the wound healing. Whereas, Deep wounds with bone and soft tissue involvement need more aggressive debridement with some involving surgery [20].

6.1.4 Foot pressure relief

The most important therapeutic principle is typically based on a quick and consistent pressure relief to promote wound healing as the weight bearing force is removed from the site of ulcer. The force redistribution is ensured by means of temporary immobilization, wearing of a protective cast or orthosis [22].

6.1.5 Wound dressings

A variety of dressing modalities are available with the advancement in the promotion of wound healing.

Dressing materials can be of various categories including natural, modified and synthetic polymers, as well as their mixtures or combinations, processed in the

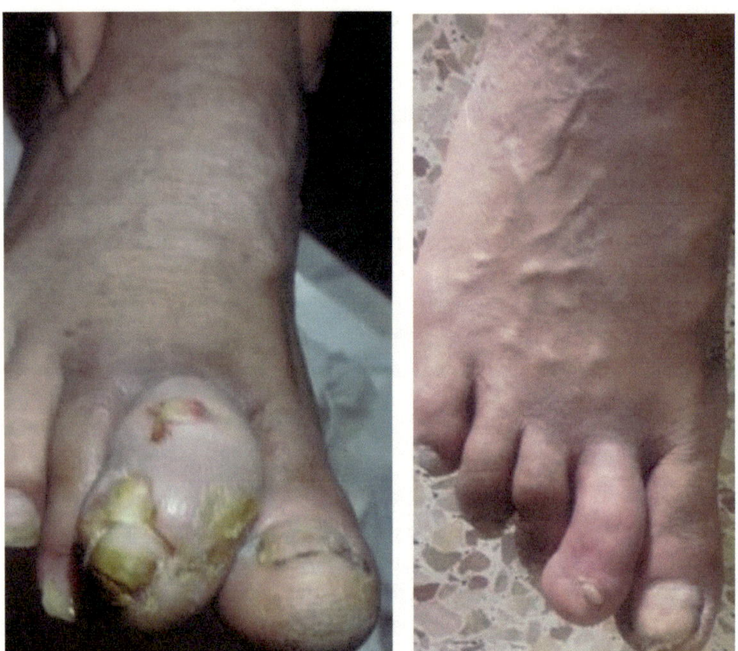

Figure 1.
Wet gangrene of the toe with osteitis. Complete healing under antibiotic treatment and MMP's inhibitor (pharysor).

form of films, foams, hydrogels and hydrocolloids. Furthermore, wound dressings can be used as medicated systems, through the delivery of healing enhancers and therapeutic substances (growth factors, peptides, drugs, stem cells and/or other bioactive substances) [2].

Randomized controlled trials [23], showed that Silver-impregnated dressings have not been shown to be more efficient in treating DFU.

Furthermore, "Moist dressings" are suggested to be more efficient than "dry dressings." [24].

According to our experience in the "Olivier Private Clinic", Sousse, Tunisia.

We noted the efficiency of Matrix Metalloproteinases (MMPs) inhibitors of natural or synthetic origin in the healing process of chronic diabetic wounds. We use mainly moist dressings with **Pharysor***, a MMPs inhibitor of natural origin, in diabetes with superficial and even with deep chronic ulcers. This agent has been found to be beneficial in improving wound healing rates (**Figures 1–4**).

Adding to that, our standard non-surgical management for DFU requires negative pressure wound therapy, close glycemic control and nutritional support with enriched oral nutritional supplement. A targeted antibiotherapy is further delivered in infected ulcers.

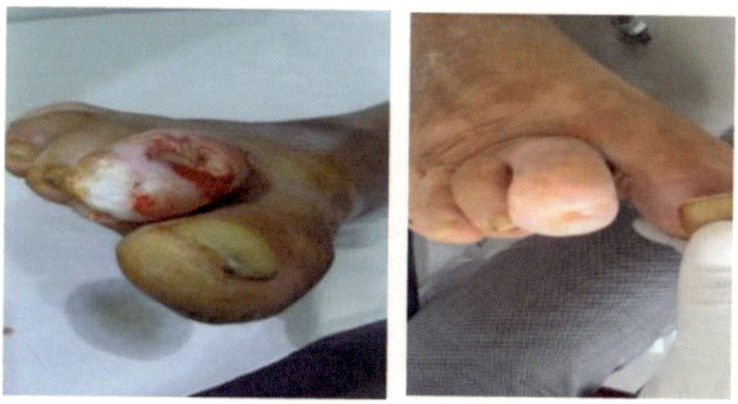

Figure 2.
Wet gangrene of the second toe with osteo-arthritis. Complete healing under antibiotic treatment and MMP's inhibitor (pharysor).

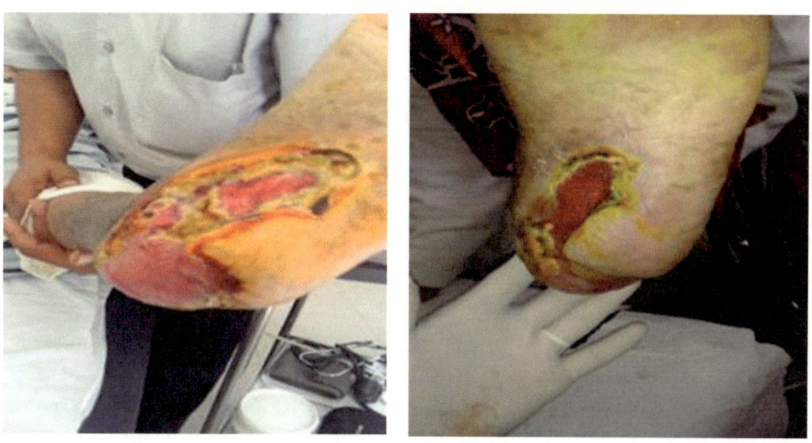

Figure 3.
Wet gangrene of the forefoot complete healing under antibiotic treatment and MMP's inhibitor (pharysor).

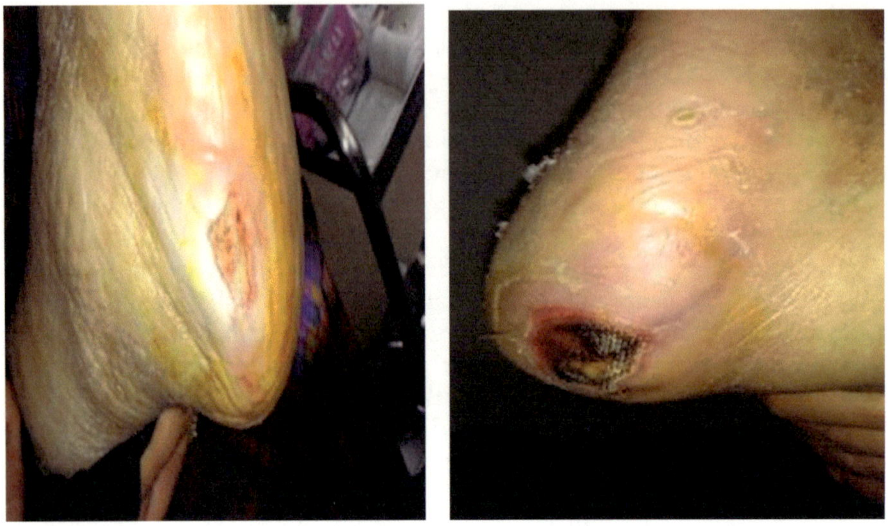

Figure 4.
Gangrene with osteitis of the calcaneus complete healing under antibiotic treatment, excision and MMP's inhibitor (pharysor).

6.2 Surgical management of DFU

Surgeons interfere in the second line and surgical approach becomes necessary when conservative and medical alternatives are not sufficient. All reconstructive surgery techniques, in particular local flaps and skin grafts, can be used depending on the location and size of the substance loss.

Furthermore, possibilities of revascularization of the lower limbs are needed to improve the chances of skin healing in case of limb ischemia.

The therapeutic decision of partial leg amputation is not systematic and should be taken as a last therapeutic option. Amputation is typically recommended for deep and chronic non healing ulcers with necrotic tissues.

7. Prevention

Preventive strategies are important to decrease the risk of repeated ulcers and amputation. Measures are mainly based on patient education and foot assessements for peripheral vascular disease and neuropathy. Furthermore, foot pressure relief with individualized orthopedic shoe provision and insole treatment is necessary in order to adapt the pressure distribution to each foot. Consequently, lesions and chronic foot ulcers may be better prevented.

8. Conclusion

Diabetic foot is a chronic complication which poses challenges in the early diagnosis and management. Paying attention to this complication is necessary during the follow-up of diabetes. The treatment is often conservative with a proper glycemic control. Management of risk factors including peripheral vascular disease, neuropathy and infection is essential to avoid serious complications leading to amputation.

Author details

Meriem Braiki[1], Mohamed Ali Khalifa[2], Bilel Faidi[3]*, Mosaab Ghannouchi[4] and Fethi Derbel[5]

1 Department of Pediatric Surgery, Regional Hospital, Sidi Bouzid, Tunisia

2 Department of Orthopedic Surgery, Sahloul University Hospital, Sousse, Tunisia

3 Department of General Surgery, Kairouan University Hospital, Sousse, Tunisia

4 Department of General Surgery, Mahdia University Hospital, Mahdia, Tunisia

5 Department of General Surgery, Oliviers Private Clinic, Sousse, Tunisia

*Address all correspondence to: fethi.derbel@gmail.com

References

[1] A.J.M. Boulton, H.Connor, Peter R, P.R.Cavanagh. The Pathway to Ulceration: Aetiopathogenesis. The Foot in Diabetes, third edition. John Wiley & Sons Ltd, Chichester.2000:19-31.

[2] Prabhu Dayal Sinwar. The diabetic foot management – Recent advance. International Journal of Surgery.2015;15:27-30.

[3] M.E. Edmonds. The diabetic foot: pathophysiology and treatment. Clinics in Endocrinology and Metabolism.1986;15(4):880-916.

[4] Maren Volmer-Thole, Ralf Lobmann. Neuropathy and Diabetic Foot Syndrome. International Journal of Molecular Sciences. Int. J. Mol. Sci. 2016:17-917.

[5] A.J.M.BoultonJ.D.Ward. Diabetic neuropathies and pain. Clinics in Endocrinology and Metabolism. 1986;15(4):917-931.

[6] P.J. Dyck, K.M. Kratz, J.L. Karnes, et al.The prevalence by staged severity of various types of diabetic neuropathy, retinopathy, and nephropathy in a population-based cohort: the Rochester Diabetic Neuropathy Study. Neurology. 1993;43: 817-824.

[7] A.J.M. Boulton, R.A. Malik, J.C. Arezzo, J.M. Sosenko. Diabetic somatic neuropathies: technical review. Diabetes Care.2004;27:1458-1486.

[8] S Syafril. Pathophysiology diabetic foot ulcer. Earth and Environmental Science. 2018.

[9] Clayton W, Elasy T A. A review of the pathophysiology, classification, and treatment of foot ulcers in diabetic patients. Clin. Diabetes.2009;27(2):52-8.

[10] Singh S, Pai R P, Yuhhui C. Diabetic foot ulcer-diagnosis and management. Clin. Res. Foot Ankle.2013;1(3):1-9.

[11] F.W. Wagner Jr. The dysvascular foot: a system for diagnosis and treatment. Foot Ankle.1981;2: 64-122.

[12] Callaghan BC, Little AA, Feldman EL and Hughes RA. Enhanced glucose control for preventing and treating diabetic neuropathy. Cochrane Database Syst Rev.2012;6.

[13] S.O. Oyibo, E.B. Jude, I. Tarawneh, H.C. Nguyen, L.B. Harkless, A.J. Boulton. A comparison of two diabetic foot ulcer classification systems: the Wagner and the University of Texas wound classification systems. Diabetes Care. 2001;24:84-8.

[14] J.J. Hurley, F.B. Hershey, A.I. Auer, H.B. Binningtoni. Noninvasive evaluation of peripheral arterial status and the physiologic approach. The Diabetic Foot, C.V. Mosby Company, London. 1983:120.

[15] Satish Chandra Mishra, Kunal C Chhatbar, Aditi Kashikar, Abha Mehndiratta.Diabetic foot. BMJ.2017;359:Supp 1.

[16] Krishnan S, Nash F, Baker N, Fowler D and Rayman G. Reduction in diabetic amputations over eleven years in a defined UK population: benefits of multi-disciplinary team work and continuous prospective audit. Diabetes Care.2008;31: 99-101.

[17] The Diabetes Control and Complications Trial Research Group. The effect of intensive treatment of diabetes on the development and progression of longterm complications in insulin-dependent diabetes mellitus. N Engl J Med.1993; 329: 977-986.

[18] Pop-Busui R, Lu J, Brooks MM, Albert S, Althouse AD, Escobedo J, et al. Impact of glycaemic control strategies on the progression of diabetic peripheral neuropathy in the bypass angioplasty

revascularisation investigation 2 Diabetes (BARI 2D) Cohort. Diabetes Care.2013;36:3208-3215.

[19] Tesfaye S, Boulton AJM and Dickenson A. Mechanisms and management of diabetic painful distal symmetrical polyneuropathy. Diabetes Care.2013;36:2456-2465.

[20] Jonathan Zhang Ming Lim, Natasha Su Lynn Ng, Cecil Thomas. Prevention and treatment of diabetic foot ulcers. Journal of the Royal Society of Medicine. 2017.110(3):104-109.

[21] Hsu CR, Chang CC, Chen YT, Lin WN and Chen MY. Organization of wound healing services: the impact on lowering the diabetes foot amputation rate in a ten-year review and the importance of early debridement. Division of Plastic Surgery, Chang Gung memorial hospital, Taiwan. Diabetes Res Clin Pract.2015;109:77-84.

[22] A.J.M. Boulton, C.I. Franks, R.P. Betts, T. Duckworth, J.D. Ward, Reduction of abnormal foot pressures in diabetic neuropathy using a new polymer insole material. Diabetes Care.1984;7:42-46.

[23] Jude EB, Apelqvist J, Spraul M and Martini J. Silver dressing study group. Prospective randomised controlled study of hydrofiber dressing containing ionic silver or calcium alginate dressing in nonischaemic diabetic foot ulcers. Diabet Med.2007;24:280-288.

[24] Dumville JC, Deschpande S, O'Meara S and Speak K. Hydrocolloid dressings for healing diabetic foot ulcers. Cochrane Database Syst.2012;2:27.

Chapter 5

Matrix Metalloproteinases (MMPs) and Diabetic Foot: Pathophysiological Findings and Recent Developments in Their Inhibitors of Natural as well as Synthetic Origin

Kirandeep Kaur, Atamjit Singh, Shivani Attri, Danish Malhotra, Aditi Verma, Neena Bedi and Preet Mohinder Singh Bedi

Abstract

Management of diabetic foot remains a major challenge for healthcare system. Though wound healing is a multiphase process and involved multiple biomarkers that acts in stepwise manner, pathophysiology diabetic foot ulcers is still not much clear and need standardization. Matrix metalloproteinases (MMPs) are often linked with non-healing characteristic of diabetic foot ulcers. They play vital roles in various phases of healing process. Major functions are removal of damaged extracellular matrix in inflammatory phase, breakdown of capillary basement membrane prior to angiogenesis and facilitation in fibroblast migration during proliferation phase. For efficient healing, these enzymes are needed in certain amount only. Imbalance of these enzymes leads to excessive degradation which has been linked with the non-healing nature of diabetic ulcers. This chapter will shed light on the role of MMP's in various phases of wound healing and the inhibitors of MMP's from natural as well as synthetic origin. It would help researchers and physicians to the understand nature of diabetic foot more clearly and design of strategies for diabetic foot management.

Keywords: diabetic foot, matrix Metalloproteinases, MMP inhibitors, wound healing, inflammation

1. Introduction

Wound healing is a complex mechanism involves cascade of inter-related events, i.e., hemostasis, inflammation, proliferation and remodeling [1]. Various skin cells including epidermal, dermal, immune and endothelial cells are involved in initiating remodeling process. In wounded are, various signaling pathways and cellular mechanisms are observed to be active at same time which are responsible for ongoing the healing process. Moreover, various cellular events such as blood clotting, fibroplasia, re-epithelization and matrix deposition along with neovascularization are also involved in the process [1–5]. Skin is the largest organ of human body and responsible to control thermoregulation, fluid imbalance and protection of other internal organs against microbes [6]. In wounds, this barrier gets disrupted and become prone to the microbial infections. The bacterial burden invades the layers beneath epidermis and also the deeper tissues associated with extracellular matrix (ECM) which worsens the wound state [7]. The matrix metalloproteinases (MMPs) are the zinc dependent proteolytic enzymes which were firstly discovered in the tadpoles having function of collagen degradation [8]. Total 24 MMPs have been reported so far having different substrate specificities and functions [9, 10]. The MMPs have been reported to be involved in cellular interactions, cell- matrix interactions by altering the levels of cytokines, growth factors and various biological fragments hidden in ECM [11–15]. MMPs indirectly modulates the cellular behavior by altering the cell surface receptors, junctional proteins and various cellular processes such as cell death and inflammation [16, 17]. MMPs play important role during microbial infection of wounds, the disrupted fragments of ECM possess antimicrobial activity which makes the MMPs to be the major component involved in healing process of wounds [18]. However, the bacteria itself are able to produce proteolytic enzymes which leads to the accumulation of degraded matrix components [19–21]. At the same time in some cases MMPs have been proven to be suitable candidate for gearing up the wound healing process [22, 23] but on other hands, several investigations reported the deregulation of these enzymes to be responsible for worsening the healing process and conversion of acute wounds to chronic wounds. This book chapter will focus on the various implications of MMPs in the chronic wounds along with their inhibitors of natural as well as synthetic origin.

2. Chronic wounds and infections

The disruption of skin barrier leads to increases susceptibility of bacterial strains to invade the wounds. The interaction of various bacteria/microbes has specificity with different matrix components turns to bacterial colonization. The bacterial colonization increases the bacterial burden in damaged wound site [24, 25]. This microbial colonization is the onset to the journey of an acute wound towards chronic wound [26, 27]. The minute to higher quantities of bacterial population is found in each and every acute wound known as contamination [28]. The quantity and the severity of these bacterial strains vary from wound to wound. If these bacterial population contains some pathogenic strains then there is a high risk of contamination turning into infection [29, 30]. Bacteria have ability to form biofilm with the help of self-secreting extracellular polymeric substances [31]. Biofilms involves the different layers of bacteria stick with each other to form thick films. These biofilms hinder the proper functioning of immune system of host [32]. The biofilms make the bacteria hard to evade from bacterial bed and delays the healing process [33]. The most prevalent bacteria found in the chronic wounds are *Staphylococcus aureus*, *Pseudomonas aeruginosa*, *Proteus mirabilis* and *Escherichia coli* which prolongs the healing process [30, 34].

3. Chronic wounds and MMPs

The elevated level of proteolytic activity of MMPs is considered as the major factor responsible for impaired wound healing [35, 36]. The MMPs have capability to degrade ECM, non-ECM components, trans-membrane proteins, cell surface receptors and diminishes the function of cytokines and growth factors by decreasing their level [37–43]. The tissue inhibitors of MMPs (TIMPs) are found to be decreased in chronic wounds that make the situation more worsen [44–47].

From the exudates of chronic wounds, it has been found that the proteolytic activity is surprisingly 116-fold higher than acute wounds. It marks the presence of MMPs in high levels [48, 49]. The plethora varies from wound to wound due to the specificity of different type of bacteria with ECM structural integrity [50, 51]. The *Staphylococcus aureus* has been found to increase the level of MMP-1 and -9 whereas *Pseudomonas aeruginosa* is known for raising the level of elastases [52, 53]. The bacterial pathogens not only target the host immune cells such as macrophages and neutrophils, but also attract the ECM matrix to release proteolytic enzymes which further mediates the release of MMPs. As in case of *Pseudomonas aeruginosa* the proteolytic enzyme thermolysin protease activates MMP-1, -8 and -9 [53]. Lipopolysaccharide derived serine proteinases activates pro-MMP-9 [54]. Different MMPs are upregulated specifically by various bacterial strains such as *Corynebacterium striatum* specifically gave rise to the level of MMP-2 and -9 and so as the other strains are specific for the modulation of MMPs [55–57].

4. MMPs and wounds

MMP family consists of 28 members, out of which 26 are expressed in humans and their homologs are found in birds, plants as well as algae also [58]. MMPs can be divided on the basis of similarity of protein fold- known an 'Clans' and on the basis of evolutionary relationships- called as 'Families'. The MMP class consists of 8 clans and almost 40 families. There are basically, two ways of classifying the MMPs, which can be described as following:

I. In accordance to the organization of the substrate specificity and homology:

    1. Collagenases (MMP-1, MMP-8, MMP-2)

    2. Gelatinases (MMP-2 and MMP-9)

    3. Stromelysins (MMP-3, MMP-10, MMP-12)

    4. Matrilysins (MMP-7, MMP-26)

    5. Membrane Type (MT) MMPs (MT-MMP-14, -15, -16, -17, -24, -25)

    6. Other MMPs (MMP-19, -20, -21, -22, -23, -27, -28)

II. In accordance to the structure of the MMPs:

    1. Archetypal MMP (type-1 collagenases)

    2. Martilysins: lacks the hemopexin domain

    3. Gelatinases: Comprised of three type II fibronectin domains

    4. MT-MMPs: Localized at the surface of cell membrane

Table 1 represents the classification of the MMPs based upon their substrate and targets. This classification provides wide range of information including their distribution in human body [59, 60].

S. no.	Type	Class	Substrates and targets	Distribution
1.	MMP-1	Collagenases	Collagen (I, II, III, VII, VIII, X), gelatin, aggrecan, nidogen, perlecan, proteoglycan link protein, serpins, tenascin C, Versican, casein, α1-antichymotrypsin, α1-antitrypsin, α1-proteinase inhibitor, IGF-BP-3 and -5, IL-1β, L-selectin, ovostatin, PAR-1, pro-TNF-α and SDF-1.	Endothelium, SMCs, fibroblasts, platelets, macrophages and varicose veins (interstitial/ fibroblast collagenase).
2.	MMP-2	Gelatinases	Collagen (I, II, III, IV, V, VII, X, XI), gelatin, aggrecan, elastin, fibronectin, laminin, nidogen, proteoglycan link protein, versican, active MMP-9 and MMP-13, FGF-R1, IGFBP-3 and -5, IL-1β, pro-TNF-α and TGF-β.	Endothelium, VSM, Adventitia, platelets, leukocytes, aortic aneurysm and varicose veins.
3.	MMP-3	Stromelysins	Collagen (II, III, IV, IX, X, XI), gelatin, aggrecan, decorin, elastin, fibronectin, laminin, nidogen, perlecan, proteoglycan, proteoglycan link protein, versican, casein, α1-antichymotrypsin, α1-proteinase inhibitor, antithrombin III, E-cadherin, fibrinogen, IGF-BP-3, L-selectin, ovostatin, pro-HB-EGF, pro-IL-1β, proMMP-1, -8, and -9, pro-TNF-α and SDF-1	Endothelium, intima, VSM, platelets, coronary artery disease, hypertension, varicose veins, synovial fibroblasts and tumor invasion.
4.	MMP-7	Matrilysins	Collagen (IV, X), gelatin, aggrecan, elastin, enactin, fibronectin, laminin, proteoglycan link protein, casein, β4 integrin, decorin, defensin, E-cadherin, Fas ligand, plasminogen, proMMP-2, -7, and -8, pro-TNF-α, syndecan and transferrin.	Endothelium, intima, VSM, uterus and varicose veins (PUMP).
5.	MMP-8	Collagenases	Collagen (I, II, III, V, VII, VIII, X), gelatin, aggrecan, elastin, fibronectin, laminin, Nidogen, α2-Antiplasmin and proMMP-8.	Macrophages and neutrophils (PMNL or neutrophil collagenase).
6.	MMP-9	Gelatinases	Collagen (IV, V, VII, X, XIV), gelatin, aggrecan, elastin, fibronectin, laminin, nidogen, proteoglycan link protein, versican, CXCL5, IL-1β, IL2-R, plasminogen, pro-TNF-α, SDF-1 and TGF-β.	Endothelium, VSM, adventitia, micro vessels, macrophages, aortic aneurysm and varicose veins.
7.	MMP-10	Stromelysins	Collagen (III, IV, V), gelatin, aggrecan, elastin, fibronectin, laminin, nidogen, Casein, proMMP-1, -8, and -10.	Atherosclerosis, uterus, preeclampsia, arthritis and carcinoma cells.
8.	MMP-11	Stromelysins	Aggrecan, fibronectin, laminin, α1-Antitrypsin, α1-proteinase inhibitor and IGF-BP-1.	Brain, uterus and angiogenesis.
9.	MMP-12	Other enzymes	Collagen IV, gelatin, elastin, fibronectin, laminin, casein and plasminogen.	SMCs, fibroblasts, macrophages and great saphenous vein.
10.	MMP-13	Collagenases	Collagen (I, II, III, IV), gelatin, aggrecan, fibronectin, laminin, perlecan, tenascin, casein, PAR-1, plasminogen activator 2, proMMP-9 and-13, and SDF-1.	SMCs, macrophages, varicose veins, pre-eclampsia and breast cancer.
11.	MMP-14	MT-MMP	Collagen (I, II, III), gelatin, aggrecan, elastin, fibrin, fibronectin, laminin, nidogen, perlecan, proteoglycan, tenascin, vitronectin, αvβ3 integrin, CD44, proMMP-2 and -13, pro-TNF-α, SDF-1, α1-proteinase inhibitor and tissue transglutaminase.	VSM, fibroblasts, platelets, brain, uterus and angiogenesis.

S. no.	Type	Class	Substrates and targets	Distribution
12.	MMP-15	MT-MMP	Collagen I, gelatin, aggrecan, fibronectin, laminin, nidogen, perlecan, tenascin, vitronectin, proMMP-2 and -13, and tissue transglutaminase	Fibroblasts, leukocytes and pre-eclampsia
13.	MMP-16	MT-MMP	Collagen I, Aggrecan, fibronectin, laminin, perlecan, vitronectin, Casein, proMMP-2 and -13	Leukocytes and angiogenesis.
14.	MMP-17	MT-MMP	Gelatin and fibrin	Brain and breast cancer.
15.	MMP-18	Collagenases	Collagen (I, II, III), gelatin and α1-Antitrypsin	Xenopus (amphibian, Xenopus collagenase), heart, lung and colon.
16.	MMP-19	Other enzymes	Collagen (I, IV), gelatin, aggrecan, fibronectin, laminin, nidogen, tenascin and casein.	Liver
17.	MMP-20	Other enzymes	Collagen (V), aggrecan, cartilage oligomeric protein and amelogenin	Tooth enamel
18.	MMP-21	Other enzymes	α1-Antitrypsin	Fibroblasts, macrophages and placenta
19.	MMP-22	Other enzymes	Gelatin	Chicken fibroblasts.
20.	MMP-23	Other enzymes	Gelatin	Ovary, testis, prostate and Other (type II) MT-MMP.
21.	MMP-24	MT-MMP	Gelatin, Chondroitin sulphate, dermatinsulfate, fibrin, fibronectin, N-cadherin and proMMP-2 and -13	Leukocytes, lung, pancreas, kidney, brain, astrocytoma and glioblastoma.
22.	MMP-25	MT-MMP	Collagen IV, gelatin, fibrin, fibronectin, proMMP-2 and α1-proteinase inhibitor	Leukocytes (leukolysin), anaplastic astrocytomas and glioblastomas.
23.	MMP-26	Matrilysins	Collagen IV, gelatin, fibrinogen, fibronectin, vitronectin, casein, β1-proteinase inhibitor, fibrin, fibronectin and proMMP-2.	Breast cancer and endometrial tumors.
24.	MMP-27	Other enzymes	—	Heart, leukocytes, macrophages, kidney, endometrium, menstruation, bone, osteoarthritis and breast cancer.
25.	MMP-28	Other enzymes	Casein	Skin and keratinocytes.

Table 1.
Distribution of MMPs in human body with their substrates and targets.

4.1 Collagenases

Collagenases are the enzymes known for their cleavage action on the bunch of extracellular components, i.e., Collagen, Aggrecan, Versican, Perlecan, etc., which are responsible for ECM accumulation. Collagenases activity has been found to be higher in chronic wounds with positively alleviated levels of MMP-1 and MMP-8 whereas the TIMP get downregulated. MMP-1 is known as collagenase-1. After the tissue rupturing, the integral proteins when coordinated with the keratinocytes alleviate the level of MMP-1. Furthermore, the MMP-1 degrades the ECM components and increases the turnover of proliferating cells at the other end of keratinocytes [61]. In the proliferation phase of wound healing the MMP-1 level is found to be high whereas the TIMPs are lower in the initial phases. On reaching the final phase of wound repair, i.e., the remodeling/re-epithelization the situation gets vice n versa. Some laminin isoforms of keratinocytes also regulate the MMPs level in various phases of wound repair [62]. In recent past several investigations report the dysregulation of MMP-1 in chronic wounds, i.e., even high level of MMP-1 is found in remodeling phase leads to damaged diabetic foot [63, 64]. The MMP/TIMP ratio is a crucial factor for repairing wounds [65]. The dermal ulcers also known as lipodermosclerosis are enriched with MMP-1 and MMP-2 associated with downregulation of TIMP-2 [66, 67]. Some immune cells stimulate the production of MMPs, i.e., collagenases and gelatinases [57, 68]. Among which the neutrophils derived MMP-8 (Collagenase-2) has been found to play an important role in pathophysiology of wounds. The upregulation of MMP-8 is majorly responsible for non-healing of wounds, i.e., for the state of chronic wounds [40, 69, 70]. On the contrary, MMP-8 has stronger affinity towards collagen-1 hence provide tensile strength to the wound tissues in the re-epithelization phase. Even in some reports MMP-8 is found to act as pro-enzyme in wound repair [71, 72]. Stromal cells derived MMP-13, collagenase-3 is reported to be highly expressed in wound site where as absence in the epidermis indicates its pivotal role in the formation of granulation tissue and extracellular matrix [63].

4.2 Gelatinases

Gelatinases, i.e., gelatinase A (MMP-2) and gelatinase B (MMP-9) have the broader specificity towards the substrates therefore leads to enhanced depletion of ECM components and retard the process of angiogenesis [6, 73]. The alleviated level of these MMPs has been found in the exudates of chronic wounds [46]. However, they possess broad specificity but an excellent substrate specificity exists between both the gelatinases. MMP-9 erodes the pro healing and other growth factors that leads to delayed in healing process however positively influence the inflammatory phase. The upregulation of MMP-9 degrades the specific biomarkers of wound healing, i.e., the vascular endothelial growth factor and dermatopontin and makes them non-functional. However MMP-2 stimulates the deterioration of laminin 332, enhance the keratinocytes migration and promotes the healing process [74–76]. The inflammatory cytokines (Interleukins; IL1-α, IL1-β, IL-2, IL-17, C reactive protein, Insulin like Growth Factors-1, Transforming Growth Factor-α) stimulates the release of protein called Neutrophil gelatinase associated lipocalin (NGAL). This NGAL activates the MMP-9 and makes the NGAL-MMP-9 complex which is considered as the underlying cause of slow healing in diabetic wounds. Diabetic wounds have been reported to be enriched with MMP-9, MMP-9-NGAL complex, NGAL and neutrophil. However, the situation gets opposite when given the insulin treatment [77–80].

4.3 Stromelysins and other MMPs

Stromelysin-1 and -2, i.e., MMP-3 and -10, respectively. MMP-3 along with collagenase-1 is found in distal end and stimulates the keratinocytes proliferation whereas MMP-10 is present in the starting edge of keratinocytes [60, 81]. MMP-3 regulates the migration of fibroblasts to the wound site resulting in wound contraction. On other hand, MMP-10 is responsible for the keratinocyte cell death and slow down the healing process. MMP-3 is a major activator of MMP-9 hence also contributing to inflammatory phase [82]. Other MMPs such as MMP-12, -7 and -14 are activated by stromal macrophages. MMP-7 interact with cyndecans and integrins to promote the skin regeneration in remodeling phase [83]. MMP-14 is majorly present in the fibroblasts on the wound bed. The level of MMP-12 gets naturally increased during inflammatory phase. These MMPs not only contribute in the cellular signaling pathways but also triggers the stimulation of other MMPs [22, 84–86].

5. MMPs in wound healing

5.1 Hemostasis

Followed by the tissue injury, the blood clotting and platelet aggregation is the former step in wound healing. The extrinsic and intrinsic system regulates the accumulation of platelets at wound site by means of coagulation factors and thrombocytes respectively [87]. The cytokines and other associated growth factors trigger the constriction of vessels which fills the voids in the wound area and lead to clot formation. The former step is followed by the vasodilation where the thrombocytes and fibroblasts like fibronectin, vitronectin and thrombospondin leads to form the provisional scaffold like wound matrix which allows the migration of keratinocytes, endothelial cells and leukocytes [88]. These platelets and leukocytes stimulate cytokines and growth factors which further assists the inflammatory process. The interleukins IL-1α, β, IL-6 and TNF-α are engaged in this process. Furthermore, the collagen synthesis is mediated by FGF-b, IGF, TGF-β and angiogenesis which get activated by FGF-B, VEGF subunit A, TGF-β and HIF-1 [89, 90]. Hemostasis is the initial phase in wound healing process and MMPs does not have any significant interference in this phase.

5.2 Proliferation and re-epithelization

The proliferation phase includes the granulation tissue to cover wound area by the strong network of vessels. Platelets are shifted to the injury site, to form the clot. Besides this, the platelets have another important function to stimulate the movement of neutrophils and macrophages to the wound site triggered by the release of platelets derived growth factors [91]. This factor is also engaged in mediating the collagenases the fibroblastic cells especially MMP-8 which have major role in tissue damage. MMP-8 are also released by neutrophils during the wound infection and assists the wound debridement and rearrangement of damaged collagen-I [92]. The synthesis of another MMPs such as MMP-1,2,3,9 are also driven by the platelets. MMP-1 and 2 has important function to control the adhesion of platelets and conglomeration [44, 88]. Moreover, MMP-9 filters the different collagen types and regulates the release of inflammatory cytokines such as IGN-γ and TGF-β. The collagen and fibroblast synthesis which in turn form the collective tissue network is also regulated by MMP-9. The new capillary formation at the wound site is also associated with movement of fibroblasts within the fibrin network which promotes angiogenesis and leads to neovascularization and re-epithelization [88]. The process of re-epithelization is also get started by the signaling pathways regulated by the endothelial and non-endothelial cells which involve various cytokines such as EGF, KGF, IGF-1 and NGF [90]. The basic component of the endothelial cells known as laminin exists in various isoforms. Among which the laminin isoform-5 have pivotal role in induction of keratinocyte migration and MMP-9 activation. Cell movement is a major role of MMP-9 hence plays an important role in re-epithelization process [93]. Another MMPs such as MMP-14 and MMP-2 breaks laminin isoform 5 and release a factor which when interacts with the epidermal growth factor (EGF) turns up the movement of cells [94, 95]. One more factor FGF-2 released by macrophages when interacts with the heparin sulphate enhances the growth of endothelial and fibroblast cells. The vascular endothelial growth factor (VEGF) released by macrophages activates the cell migration and proliferation of keratinocytes and endothelial cells which include MMP-1, 2, 9 and 13 hence play a major role in wound healing [96, 97].

5.3 Matrix formation and remodeling

The final stage of wound healing is remodeling phase. It involves the upregulation of collagen turnover but decline in proliferation of fibroblast [98]. Moreover, the keratinocytes reach fibrin clot by crossing granulation tissue matrix [99]. The collagen-I replacement with collagen type III indicates the maturation of wound [100, 101]. However, in the early phase of remodeling phase fibronectin and fibroblasts are get displaced by collagen type I and III and proteoglycans which in turn enhances the tensile strength and integrity of wound matrix [102]. The level of myofibroblast and blood vessels get increased while reaching the end of this phase and high density of these two leads to the closure of wound [63, 103].

5.4 Proteolysis in wound repair

Many processes in wound healing such as keratinocyte migration, angiogenesis and re-epithelization are generally followed by the extra cellular matrix (ECM) degradation [104]. The MMPs are majorly involved in this proteolytic degradation. MMP-19 and 28 are present in keratinocytes of basal stratum and superbasals [105]. Moreover, MMP-19 is also found in the hair follicles, endothelial cells, arteries and veins [106]. MMP-1 expression is found to be upregulated in dermis part of the wounds where basal membrane is destroyed and promotes re-epithelization process and triggers the binding of keratinocytes with type-1 collagen [65]. Collagen type I is known to upregulate the level of MMP-1 whereas collagen type III and other basement proteins do not promote the MMP-1 synthesis. MMP-1 activates $\alpha1\beta2$ integrin to synthesize collagen type-1 [16]. The MMP1- $\alpha1\beta2$ complex enhances the migration of keratinocytes therefore boost up the re-epithelization process [107]. During the process of basement membrane formation followed by re-epithelization, MMP-1 expression gets knockdown by the cellular junctions of basal membrane proteins [16, 108]. Moreover, MMP-13 which is mainly present in the dermis along with MMP-1 regulates the fibroblast proliferation mediated by matrix shrinkage and matrix stiffness [109, 110]. MMP-8 stored in cellular granules are secreted when get activated by macrophages [111]. The overexpression of MMP-8 is found in the damaged wounds. MMP-13 downregulation is balanced by MMP-8 which slow down the healing process by improper infiltration of neutrophils, improper re-epithelization and constant inflammatory syndrome [111, 112]. As given in the classification section the stromelysins such as MMP-3 and MMP-10 are present in the epidermal cells i.e. proliferating keratinocytes. These MMPs especially MMP-3 has major role in disruption of fibrin containing provisional matrix and formation of new basal matrix after remodeling [113]. This process is majorly carried out by cytokines and other growth factors such as FGF-b and HB-EGF [114]. Furthermore, the MMP-9 has also an important role in final phase that shaping the epidermal layer at the end during wound repair. In addition, MMP-2, -9, -19 and MT1-MMP are stored and released by the endothelial cells [115]. Among which MMP-2 and -9 have pivotal role in degradation of mature blood vessels and sprouting/growth of new blood vessels by activating angiogenesis related growth factors and cytokines [86, 89, 116, 117]. MT1-MMP possess proteolytic activity against mature collagen and fibrin by crossing the thick network of fibrin proteins in stroma of damaged tissues [118]. Whereas, MMP-19 is involved in growth process of endothelial cells, epithelial cells, fibroblast cells and small vasculature within macrophages [119].

The wounds that persist more than 4–6 weeks are generally recognized as chronic wounds [120]. Wounds such as venous leg ulcers [72, 121], diabetic foot ulcers [122, 123] and that caused due to pressure [66] are considered as chronic or delayed wounds. Some wounds which appears to be acute at initial stages but may turns to chronic one while reaching the final phase of healing are also categorized under chronic wounds. Main examples of these types of wounds are surgical wounds and traumatic wounds. These chronic wounds are specifically characterized by the altered levels on MMPs.

Abnormal structural integrity of fibrin network, increased tendon rigidity and altered volume and level of biochemical substances indicates the delayed and chronic wounds [124]. Proteolytic activity of MMPs has major impact on healing process of chronic wounds. Besides this MMP-3 and MMP-13 along with MMP-9 are actively found in the normal as well as diabetic foot ulcers. Where MMP-3 and MMP-9 have been upregulated, MMP-3 has been found to be knockdown in chronic wounds. The overexpression of MMP-13 and MMP-9 is associated with high glucose concentration at wound site [125]. The imbalance between MMP and TIMP level is a major cause of hyperglycemia, hyperlipidemia and hypertension during the condition of chronic wounds/diabetic ulcers [126, 127]. In the state of chronic wounds, the migration of inflammatory cells is followed by imbalanced fibroblast clotting which lead to secrete the ECM proteins. Meanwhile, MMPs have been found to increase the fibroblast proliferation and collagen degradation via TGF-β1 signaling [127, 128]. Higher production of gelatinases has been observed in the diabetic wounds. Conclusively MMPs in this state are associated with degradation of ECM components but at the same time are also responsible for the recovery of traumatic wounds by regenerating the capillary and blood vessels at the respective site [129].

6. Levels of MMPs in diabetic wounds

In the state of diabetic wounds, the glucose level is significantly higher [130]. Elevated levels of MMPs have been found in these wounds because of oxidative stress and end products of glycation which may lead to diabetic peripheral arterial disease [61, 131]. Degradation of ECM due to MMPs especially MMP-1, -2 and -9 turn these diabetic wounds to get more worse [132]. The mismatch between the extent of degradation and repairing of ECM is a critical factor to cause delay in wound healing process i.e. chronic wounds. Therefore, it necessitates the ECM components to be in controlled condition for boosting up the healing process [131]. Any other disease condition in diabetic ulcer may worsen the healing process due to imbalanced availability of cytokines and other growth factors needed for the healing of wounds [133, 134]. In each phase of diabetic wound repair, i.e., hemostasis, inflammation, proliferation and remodeling there has been altered expression of MMPs [135]. Epithelial remodeling is associated with raised levels of MMP-1, -8, -9 and downregulation of TIMPs. The fibronectin degradation is majorly carried out by MMP-9 which leads to cell migration and proliferation [136]. MMP-1, -8 and -9 have been reported to be upregulated in the venous wounds due to absence of TIMP [73, 81]. Patients with metabolic syndrome have been found to be overly expressed with MMP-2 and -9 in their serum sample. The mutations in the gene expression of MMP-9 can also be a cause for delayed healing. Increased expression of MMP-9, TNF-α and other growth factors in diabetic foot ulcers has been found and concluded that they could be linked with slow-to-heal ulcers in diabetics and therefore a target for new therapeutic management [137].

7. Therapeutical targeting of MMPs

7.1 Synthetic approaches

MMPs has pivotal role in diabetic wounds hence they are the major target for the researchers. MMPs possess high resemblance in their structural morphology therefore it is difficult to target specifically one MMP at the time especially when they fall under same category such as gelatinase-A and gelatinase-B [138, 139]. Moreover, MMP-8 has been found to boost up healing in diabetic wounds in absence of MMP-9 and vice versa which necessitates the specific inhibition of MMP-9 without having any interaction with MMP-8. There are many broad spectrum MMP inhibitors (MMPI) which have been already investigated for the purpose but we need more selective therapeutics over the existing one [140]. Many small structural molecules have been discovered yet to target the same. In an investigation, it has been reported that the racemic mixture, i.e., (R, S)-ND-336 possess 55-fold more activity than the R or S isomer alone to target MMP-9 specifically than MMP-8 [74]. Moreover, based upon the Ki values the R isomer has been reported to be 10-fold more potent than the S isomer for selective inhibition of MMP-9 [141]. As it has been known that the synthetic molecule (R, S)-ND-336 falls under thiirane class, its structural ring gets unlatched and produce thiolate which gets interacted with the zinc ion within MMP-9 and inhibit its function. Reversal of the given process is very slow therefore it shows long lasting retention time. R-ND-336 has been investigated to be more effective than FDA approved drug becaplermin for the respective purpose [141]. Enhanced specificity for inhibition of MMPs can be obtained by using antibody approach. In the recent past, GS-5745 is an antibody being investigated for specific inhibition of MMP-9. It has dual mechanism to act on i.e. by interacting and hindering the active site of MMP-9 and another one is to cleave the MMP-3 zymogen which is involved in activation of MMP-9 [142–145]. Moreover, another two antibodies being investigated under the clinical trials are SSDS-3 and REGA-3G12 have been observed to possess selective inhibition against MMP-9 [146, 147]. Furthermore, the above antibodies have been more explored for the cancer targets hence there are many future possibilities to explore the wound healing potential of the above candidates [148]. Wound dressings are being commonly used for the purpose of healing and controlling the exudate secretion [149]. Many MMP inhibitors have been used to incorporate into these wound dressings. But these inhibitors are generally found to be non-specific, i.e., the broad-spectrum inhibitors. Most commonly used MMP-inhibitors in wound healing are bisphosphonates [150]. Another hypothesis involves the use of atelocollagen type I to be used along with 4-vinyl-benzyl chloride to specifically inhibit the MMPs present in wound exudates [151]. In addition, another clinical candidate GM-6001 exploited as wound dressing has broad spectrum activity but found to be less effecting in healing diabetic wounds than the therapeutics having specific inhibitors against MMPs [152]. RNA is a basic nucleotide to synthesize gene encoding MMPs [153]. So, the therapies being approached to inhibit RNA which in turn inhibit the MMPs at gene level have the high potential to heal the diabetic wounds than other therapeutics [154]. But the major obstacle is to deliver the siRNA to the target site [155–157]. Therefore, to overcome this, the star shaped cationic polymer such as cyclodextrins have been reported to be used for the purpose as they have very low toxicity [158]. Furthermore, β-CD-(D3)7/MMP-9-siRNA has been found in an investigation to inhibit MMP-9 in the diabetic wounds where MMPs level is quite high due to TIMP knockdown which in turn promotes the healing process. These siRNAs are supposed to be taken by the fibroblasts on wound site [159, 160]. But when the siRNA was used alone in a further study it has been found to cause liver and kidney toxicity [161]. In addition, the miRNA-139 and miRNA-335 has been reported to possess an excellent potential in healing the diabetic wounds via inhibiting MMP-9 [162].

7.2 MMPs inhibitors of natural origin

Natural products have huge resource of biologically active molecules and provided large number of biologically active compounds to clinical practice for treatment of wide range of diseases and disorders. Considering capability of natural products in drug development, wide range of researchers across the globe has screened numerous constituents from natural sources for MMPs modulation activity. Major bioactive constituents (**Figure 1**) from natural sources with MMP modulation potential has been discussed below.

Withaferin A (3-azido Withaferin A) a naturally derived steroidal lactone from plant *Withania somnifera*, exhibits various pharmacological activities. *In vitro* studies revealed that withaferin A inhibit MMP-2 by up regulating the expression of pro-apoptotic protein par-4. Stimulation of par-4 by withaferin A enhances apoptosis by extrinsic pathway of apoptosis by activating FADD-caspase-8-caspase-3 in dose dependent manner [163]. Cantharidin is a natural compound obtained from *Mylabris phalerata* and showed remarkable inhibition of cell migration and invasiveness by suppressing MMP-2 and MMP-9 through affecting their upstream markers such as NF-κB, c-Jun and AP-1 in A375.S2 cells based wound healing and matrigel chamber invasion assays. Cantharidin exerts anti-cell migration and anti-invasiveness property by suppressing MMP-2 and MMP-9 via modulating their upstream markers such as NF-κB, c-Jun and AP-1. Cantharidin also down regulate the expression of NF-κB, p65 and proteins involved in PI3K-Akt (PI3K, ERK1/2, Rock1 and FAK) and MAPK (p38, ERK and JNK) signaling cascade [164]. Celastrol is another phytoconstituent of *Tripterygium wilfordii* having anti-proliferative activity. Celastrol inhibit metastasis and invasiveness of ovarian cancer cells (SKOV3 and OVCAR-3) by knockdown the expression of NF-κB/MMP-9. NF-κB modulates IκBα degradation, p65 translocation blocking and MMP-9 suppression [165]. Gallic acid has been proved to inhibit cell metastasis and invasiveness in PC-3 cells by degrading expressions of MMP-2 and MMP-9 otherwise they degrade the ECM and delayed wound healing. Gallic acid has been also observed to activate the TIMP-1 which is natural regulator of MMP-2 [166]. Ginsenoside Rd is obtained from *Panax ginseng* leaf which increases proliferation, migration and shows protective effect in human dermal fibroblast (HDFs) and keratinocyte progenitor cells which enhances healing of skin wound. Being a steroidal moiety it easily permeate to cell membrane and enhance healing of skin both in laser burn and excision wound by increasing expression of CREB, cAMP along with reducing expression of MMP-1 [167]. Lycorine a natural compound widely distributed in plant family Amaryllidaceae. Lycorine shows antimigratory effect in HepG2 cells by reducing the expression of MMP-2 and MMP-9. Lycorine increase polymerized F-actin by blocking the normal turnover of the actin cytoskeleton and a loss of depolymerized G-actin. The activation of ROCK1 in cells pre-treated with lycorine shows decrease in expression of cofilin, cyclinA, cyclin B1, cdc2, MMP-9 and MMP-2

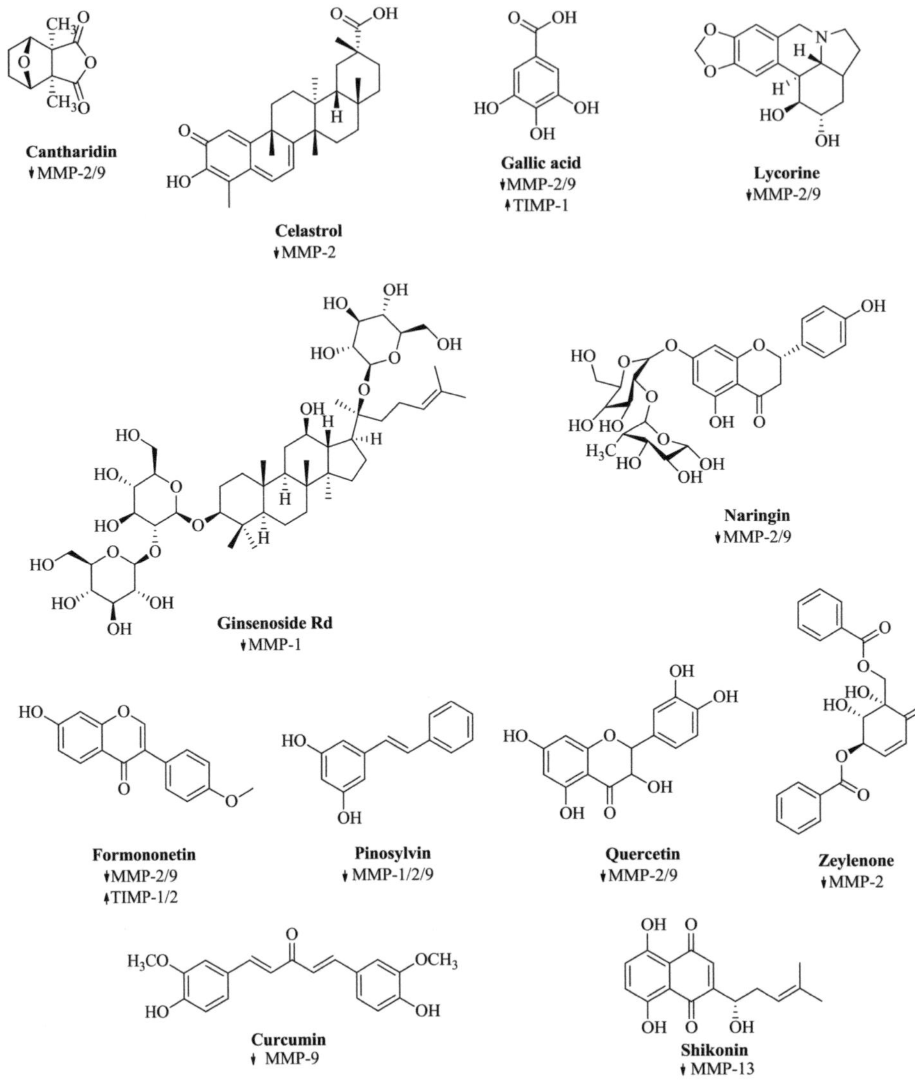

Figure 1.
Various MMP inhibitors of natural origin.

which shows lycorine inhibiting cell proliferation and migration in HepG2 cells via inhibition of ROCK1/cofilin-induced actin dynamics [168]. Naringin is a natural flavonoid present in citrus fruits. Treatment of naringin reduce the expression of p-ERK and p-JNK which are molecular markers involved in MAPK signaling pathway in turn reduce the expression of MMP-2 and MMP-9 [169]. Pinosylvin is a natural compound present in *Pinus* species. Pinosylvin downregulate the expressions of MMP-1, MMP-2 and MMP-9 in human fibrosarcoma HT1080 cells. Quercetin is another well-known inhibitor of MMP-2 and MMP-9 [170]. Platycodin D from *Platycodon grandiflorum* exhibit anti-invasive and antimetastatic activity in human breast cancer cells (MDA-MB-231). It inhibit cell invasion by down regulating the Mrna expression of MMP-9 [171]. Formononetin is a natural compound found in *Astragalus membranaceus, Trifolium pratense, Glycyrrhiza glabra* and *Pueraria lobata.* It shows inhibitory effect on the breast cancer cells progression, migration and invasiveness by suppressing the effect of MMP-2 and MMP-9 along with upregulating the expression of matrix metalloproteinase inhibitors such as TIMP-1 and TIMP-2 [172]. Zeylenone is natural oxide with anticancer activity. In the present study, Zey is reported to have anti-cancer activity against prostate cancer. Zeylenone has been reported to suppress the expression of MMP-2, MMP-9 and upregulate the expression of TIMP-1 and collagen-1 in DU145 cells [173]. Curcumin is a natural compound extracted from plant *Curcuma longa* (Zingiberaceae). Curcumin possesses anti-oxidant, anti-inflammatory and anti-cancer activity and along with wound healing property. The mechanism of curcumin behind wound healing is the lowering the expression of TNF-α and increased proportion of α-SMA and collagen in fibroblast. Matrix metalloproteinase especially MMP-9 helpful in tissue migration and remodeling and someway helpful in normal wound healing. Curcumin treated cells negatively regulate the expression of MMP-9 and reduced the expression of TNF-α which positively modulate MMP-9. Curcumin also regulate the expression of NF-κB induce by TNF-α. Thus curcumin enhances wound healing activity by downregulating expression of MMP-9 and increase value of collagen by regulating expression of NF-κB induce by TNF-α in fibroblasts [174]. Shikonin is a natural component presents in *Lithospermum erythrorhizon* which exhibit decent wound healing property. Shikonin has been proved for its inhibitory effect on migration and invasiveness of U87 and U251cells by inhibiting the expression of MMP-2 and MMP-9 [175, 176].

8. Conclusion

From the ancient past wound healing has known to be a complicated topic as it involves many complex and unclear mechanisms. Moreover, wound healing process in diabetes like state get delay and more worsen. In the recent past various MMPs have been found to play a key role in the healing of diabetic foot. Structurally, it mainly has zinc on its active site. Furthermore, it is categorized in various types based upon the different substrate it cleaves, i.e., collagenases, gelatinases, stromelysins and various other MMPs. Also, the modulation of expression of various MMPs significantly alters the healing process. In addition, TGF-β has been reported to be the signaling pathway for MMPs to act upon for healing of chronic wounds. Moreover, different phases of wound repair involve alteration in level of various MMPs. Among various MMPs, MMP-9 has been widely discussed and investigated enzyme in the recent past and has also been considered as major culprit in altering the healing rate. The overexpression of various MMPs extends the time of healing or may devastate the condition. Therefore, various MMP inhibitors either of natural or synthetic origin have been explored for the purpose. Most of these candidates are under clinical trial and has proven to be very selective and effective for healing chronic wounds. Besides the wound healing MMPs possess therapeutic effectiveness for various other diseases. In future, there are various possibilities to explore and unlash various mechanisms of MMPs for chronic wound healing.

Acknowledgements

Authors are grateful to the University Grants Commission for providing NFOBC to Atamjit Singh. The authors are also thankful to Guru Nanak Dev University, Amritsar for providing various facilities to carry out the work.

Conflict of interest

The authors confirm that this chapter content has no conflicts of interest.

Author details

Kirandeep Kaur[1†], Atamjit Singh[1*†], Shivani Attri[2], Danish Malhotra[1], Aditi Verma[1], Neena Bedi[1*] and Preet Mohinder Singh Bedi[1*]

1 Department of Pharmaceutical Sciences, Guru Nanak Dev University, Amritsar, Punjab, India

2 Department of Botanical and Environmental Sciences, Guru Nanak Dev University, Amritsar, Punjab, India

*Address all correspondence to: atamjitpharma.rsh@gndu.ac.in, neena.pharma@gndu.ac.in and bedi_preet@yahoo.com

† Both sharing co-first authorship.

References

[1] Diegelmann RF. From the selected works of Robert F. Diegelmann Ph. D. Frontiers in Bioscience. 2004;**9**:283-289

[2] Shaw TJ, Martin P. Wound repair at a glance. Journal of Cell Science. 2009;**122**(18):3209-3213

[3] Yamaguchi Y, Yoshikawa K. Cutaneous wound healing: An update. The Journal of Dermatology. 2001;**28**(10):521-534

[4] Martin P. Wound healing--aiming for perfect skin regeneration. Science. 1997;**276**(5309):75-81

[5] Schultz GS, Davidson JM, Kirsner RS, Bornstein P, Herman IM. Dynamic reciprocity in the wound microenvironment. Wound Repair and Regeneration. 2011;**19**(2):134-148

[6] Cooper S. The biology of the skin. Journal of the Royal Society of Medicine. 2002;**95**:109

[7] Yager DR, Zhang LY, Liang HX, Diegelmann RF, Cohen IK. Elevated matrix metalloproteinase levels and activity compared to surgical wound fluids. Journal of Investigative Dermatology. 1996;**107**(5):743-748

[8] Gross J, Lapiere CM. Collagenolytic activity in amphibian tissues: A tissue culture assay. Proceedings of the National Academy of Sciences of the United States of America. 1962;**48**(6):1014

[9] Puente XS, Sánchez LM, Overall CM, López-Otín C. Human and mouse proteases: A comparative genomic approach. Nature Reviews. Genetics. 2003;**4**(7):544-558

[10] Fanjul-Fernández M, Folgueras AR, Cabrera S, López-Otín C. Matrix metalloproteinases: Evolution, gene regulation and functional analysis in mouse models. Biochimica et Biophysica Acta (BBA)-Molecular Cell Research. 2010;**1803**(1):3-19

[11] Levi E, Fridman R, Miao HQ, Ma YS, Yayon A, Vlodavsky I. Matrix metalloproteinase 2 releases active soluble ectodomain of fibroblast growth factor receptor 1. Proceedings of the National Academy of Sciences. 1996;**93**(14):7069-7074

[12] Preece G, Murphy G, Ager A. Metalloproteinase-mediated regulation of L-selectin levels on leucocytes. Journal of Biological Chemistry. 1996;**271**(20):11634-11640

[13] Suzuki M, Raab G, Moses MA, Fernandez CA, Klagsbrun M. Matrix metalloproteinase-3 releases active heparin-binding EGF-like growth factor by cleavage at a specific juxtamembrane site. Journal of Biological Chemistry. 1997;**272**(50):31730-31737

[14] Rundhaug JE. Matrix metalloproteinases and angiogenesis. Journal of Cellular and Molecular Medicine. 2005;**9**(2):267-285

[15] Solomonov I, Zehorai E, Talmi-Frank D, Wolf SG, Shainskaya A, Zhuravlev A, et al. Distinct biological events generated by ECM proteolysis by two homologous collagenases. Proceedings of the National Academy of Sciences. 2016;**113**(39):10884-10889

[16] Sternlicht MD, Werb Z. How matrix metalloproteinases regulate cell behavior. Annual Review of Cell and Developmental Biology. 2001;**17**(1):463-516

[17] Chen Q, Jin M, Yang F, Zhu J, Xiao Q, Zhang L. Matrix metalloproteinases: Inflammatory regulators of cell behaviors in vascular formation and remodeling. Mediators of Inflammation. 2013;**2013**:928315

[18] Brennan EP, Reing J, Chew D, Myers-Irvin JM, Young EJ, Badylak SF. Antibacterial activity within degradation products of biological scaffolds composed of extracellular matrix. Tissue Engineering. 2006;**12**(10):2949-2955

[19] Suleman L. Extracellular bacterial proteases in chronic wounds: A potential therapeutic target? Advances in Wound Care. 2016;**5**(10):455-463

[20] Maeda H, Molla A. Pathogenic potentials of bacterial proteases. Clinica Chimica Acta. 1989;**185**(3):357-367

[21] Wong W, Wijeyewickrema LC, Kennan RM, Reeve SB, Steer DL, Reboul C, et al. S1 pocket of a bacterially derived subtilisin-like protease underpins effective tissue destruction. Journal of Biological Chemistry. 2011;**286**(49):42180-42187

[22] Ravanti L, Kähäri VM. Matrix metalloproteinases in wound repair. International Journal of Molecular Medicine. 2000;**6**(4):391-798

[23] Steffensen B, Häkkinen L, Larjava H. Proteolytic events of wound-healing—Coordinated interactions among matrix metalloproteinases (MMPs), integrins, and extracellular matrix molecules. Critical Reviews in Oral Biology and Medicine. 2001;**12**(5):373-398

[24] Lähteenmäki K, Virkola R, Sarén A, Emödy L, Korhonen TK. Expression of plasminogen activator Pla of *Yersinia pestis* enhances bacterial attachment to the mammalian extracellular matrix. Infection and Immunity. 1998;**66**(12):5755-5762

[25] Chauhan N, Wrobel A, Skurnik M, Leo JC. *Yersinia adhesins*: An arsenal for infection. PROTEOMICS–Clinical Applications. 2016;**10**(9-10):949-963

[26] Stevens DL, Bisno AL, Chambers HF, Dellinger EP, Goldstein EJ, Gorbach SL, et al. Practice guidelines for the diagnosis and management of skin and soft tissue infections: 2014 update by the Infectious Diseases Society of America. Clinical Infectious Diseases. 2014;**59**(2):e10-e52

[27] McMenemy K. Skin and soft tissue infections. Physician Assistant Clinics. 2017;**2**(2):165-176

[28] Edwards R, Harding KG. Bacteria and wound healing. Current Opinion in Infectious Diseases. 2004;**17**(2):91-96

[29] Cooper R, Lawrence JC. The isolation and identification of bacteria from wounds. Journal of Wound Care. 1996;**5**(7):335-340

[30] Bessa LJ, Fazii P, Di Giulio M, Cellini L. Bacterial isolates from infected wounds and their antibiotic susceptibility pattern: Some remarks about wound infection. International Wound Journal. 2015;**12**(1):47-52

[31] Flemming HC, Wingender J. The biofilm matrix. Nature Reviews Microbiology. 2010;**8**(9):623-633

[32] Metcalf DG, Bowler PG. Biofilm delays wound healing: A review of the evidence. Burns & Trauma. 2013;**1**(1):5-12

[33] Attinger C, Wolcott R. Clinically addressing biofilm in chronic wounds. Advances in Wound Care. 2012;**1**(3):127-132

[34] Dowd SE, Sun Y, Secor PR, Rhoads DD, Wolcott BM, James GA, et al. Survey of bacterial diversity in chronic wounds using pyrosequencing, DGGE, and full ribosome shotgun sequencing. BMC Microbiology. 2008;**8**(1):43

[35] Rayment EA, Upton Z. Finding the culprit: A review of the influences of proteases on the chronic wound

environment. The International Journal of Lower Extremity Wounds. 2009;**8**(1):19-27

[36] Trengove NJ, Stacey MC, Macauley S, Bennett N, Gibson J, Burslem F, et al. Analysis of the acute and chronic wound environments: The role of proteases and their inhibitors. Wound Repair and Regeneration. 1999;**7**(6):442-452

[37] Shapiro SD. Matrix metalloproteinase degradation of extracellular matrix: biological consequences. Current Opinion in Cell Biology. 1998;**10**(5):602-608

[38] Yue J, Zhang K, Chen J. Role of integrins in regulating proteases to mediate extracellular matrix remodeling. Cancer Microenvironment. 2012;**5**(3):275-283

[39] Bullen EC, Longaker MT, Updike DL, Benton R, Ladin D, Hou Z, et al. Tissue inhibitor of metalloproteinases-1 is decreased and activated gelatinases are increased in chronic wounds. Journal of Investigative Dermatology. 1995;**104**(2):236-240

[40] Schultz GS, Wysocki A. Interactions between extracellular matrix and growth factors in wound healing. Wound Repair and Regeneration. 2009;**17**(2):153-162

[41] Krishnaswamy VR, Manikandan M, Munirajan AK, Vijayaraghavan D, Korrapati PS. Expression and integrity of dermatopontin in chronic cutaneous wounds: A crucial factor in impaired wound healing. Cell and Tissue Research. 2014;**358**(3):833-841

[42] Mast BA, Schultz GS. Interactions of cytokines, growth factors, and proteases in acute and chronic wounds. Wound Repair and Regeneration. 1996;**4**(4):411-420

[43] Kryczka J, Stasiak M, Dziki L, Mik M, Dziki A, Cierniewski CS. Matrix metalloproteinase-2 cleavage of the β1 integrin ectodomain facilitates colon cancer cell motility. Journal of Biological Chemistry. 2012;**287**(43):36556-36566

[44] Armstrong DG, Jude EB. The role of matrix metalloproteinases in wound healing. Journal of the American Podiatric Medical Association. 2002;**92**(1):12-18

[45] Yanhan R, Guosheng G, Min Y, Driver VR. Role of matrix metalloproteinases in chronic wound healing: Diagnostic and therapeutic implications. Chinese Medical Journal. 2014;**127**(8):1572-1581

[46] Lobmann R, Ambrosch A, Schultz G, Waldmann K, Schiweck S, Lehnert H. Expression of matrix-metalloproteinases and their inhibitors in the wounds of diabetic and non-diabetic patients. Diabetologia. 2002;**45**(7):1011-1016

[47] Robson MC. The role of growth factors in the healing of chronic wounds. Wound Repair and Regeneration. 1997;**5**(1):12-17

[48] Gaffney J, Solomonov I, Zehorai E, Sagi I. Multilevel regulation of matrix metalloproteinases in tissue homeostasis indicates their molecular specificity in vivo. Matrix Biology. 2015;**44**:191-199

[49] Tarnuzzer RW, Schultz GS. Biochemical analysis of acute and chronic wound environments. Wound Repair and Regeneration. 1996;**4**(3):321-325

[50] Santala A, Saarinen J, Kovanen P, Kuusela P. Activation of interstitial collagenase, MMP-1, by *Staphylococcus aureus* cells having surface-bound plasmin: A novel role of plasminogen receptors of bacteria. FEBS Letters. 1999;**461**(3):153-156

[51] Calander AM, Starckx S, Opdenakker G, Bergin P,

Quiding-Järbrink M, Tarkowski A. Matrix metalloproteinase-9 (gelatinase B) deficiency leads to increased severity of *Staphylococcus aureus*-triggered septic arthritis. Microbes and Infection. 2006;**8**(6):1434-1439

[52] Schmidtchen A, Holst E, Tapper H, Björck L. Elastase-producing *Pseudomonas aeruginosa* degrade plasma proteins and extracellular products of human skin and fibroblasts, and inhibit fibroblast growth. Microbial Pathogenesis. 2003;**34**(1):47-55

[53] Okamoto T, Akaike T, Suga M, Tanase S, Horie H, Miyajima S, et al. Activation of human matrix metalloproteinases by various bacterial proteinases. Journal of Biological Chemistry. 1997;**272**(9):6059-6066

[54] Min D, Moore AG, Bain MA, Breit SN, Lyons JG. Activation of macrophage promatrix metalloproteinase-9 by lipopolysaccharide-associated proteinases. The Journal of Immunology. 2002;**168**(5):2449-2455

[55] DeCarlo AA Jr, Windsor LJ, Bodden MK, Harber GJ, Birkedal-Hansen B, Birkedal-Hansen H. Activation and novel processing of matrix metalloproteinases by a thiol-proteinase from the oral anaerobe *Porphyromonas gingivalis*. Journal of Dental Research. 1997;**76**(6):1260-1270

[56] Oggioni MR, Memmi G, Maggi T, Chiavolini D, Iannelli F, Pozzi G. Pneumococcal zinc metalloproteinase ZmpC cleaves human matrix metalloproteinase 9 and is a virulence factor in experimental pneumonia. Molecular Microbiology. 2003;**49**(3):795-805

[57] Serra R, Grande R, Buffone G, Molinari V, Perri P, Perri A, et al. Extracellular matrix assessment of infected chronic venous leg ulcers: Role of metalloproteinases and inflammatory cytokines. International Wound Journal. 2016;**13**(1):53-58

[58] Wang X, Khalil RA. Matrix metalloproteinases, vascular remodeling, and vascular disease. In: Advances in Pharmacology. 2018;**81**:241-330

[59] Li W, Saji S, Sato F, Noda M, Toi M. Potential clinical applications of matrix metalloproteinase inhibitors and their future prospects. The International Journal of Biological Markers. 2013;**28**(2):117-130

[60] Gueders MM, Foidart JM, Noel A, Cataldo DD. Matrix metalloproteinases (MMPs) and tissue inhibitors of MMPs in the respiratory tract: Potential implications in asthma and other lung diseases. European Journal of Pharmacology. 2006;**533**(1-3):133-144

[61] Martins VL, Caley M, O'Toole EA. Matrix metalloproteinases and epidermal wound repair. Cell and Tissue Research. 2013;**351**(2):255-268

[62] Parks WC. Matrix metalloproteinases in repair. Wound Repair and Regeneration. 1999;**7**(6):423-432

[63] Saarialho-Kere UK. Patterns of matrix metalloproteinase and TIMP expression in chronic ulcers. Archives of Dermatological Research. 1998;**290**(1):S47-S54

[64] McCawley LJ, Matrisian LM. Matrix metalloproteinases: They're not just for matrix anymore! Current Opinion in Cell Biology. 2001;**13**(5):534-540

[65] Sudbeck BD, Pilcher BK, Welgus HG, Parks WC. Induction and repression of collagenase-1 by keratinocytes is controlled by distinct components of different extracellular matrix compartments. Journal of Biological Chemistry. 1997;**272**(35):22103-22110

[66] Barone EJ, Yager DR, Pozez AL, Olutoye OO, Crossland MC, Diegelmann RF, et al. Interleukin-1alpha and collagenase activity are elevated in chronic wounds. Plastic and Reconstructive Surgery. 1998;**102**(4):1023-1027

[67] Muller M, Trocme C, Lardy B, Morel F, Halimi S, Benhamou PY. Matrix metalloproteinases and diabetic foot ulcers: The ratio of MMP-1 to TIMP-1 is a predictor of wound healing. Diabetic Medicine. 2008;**25**(4):419-426

[68] Herouy YA, Nockowski PI, Schöpf ER, Norgauer JO. Lipodermatosclerosis and the significance of proteolytic remodeling in the pathogenesis of venous ulceration. International Journal of Molecular Medicine. 1999;**3**(5):511-516

[69] Herouy Y, Pornschlegel G, Stetter C, Grenz H, Schöpf E, Norgauer J, et al. Lipodermatosclerosis is characterized by elevated expression and activation of matrix metalloproteinases: Implications for venous ulcer formation. Journal of Investigative Dermatology. 1998;**111**(5):822-827

[70] Percival SL, Finnegan S, Donelli G, Vuotto C, Rimmer S, Lipsky BA. Antiseptics for treating infected wounds: Efficacy on biofilms and effect of pH. Critical Reviews in Microbiology. 2016;**42**(2):293-309

[71] Harris IR, Yee KC, Walters CE, Cunliffe WJ, Kearney JN, Wood EJ, et al. Cytokine and protease levels in healing and non-healing chronic venous leg ulcers. Experimental Dermatology. 1995;**4**(6):342-349

[72] Nwomeh BC, Liang HX, Cohen IK, Yager DR. MMP-8 is the predominant collagenase in healing wounds and nonhealing ulcers. Journal of Surgical Research. 1999;**81**(2):189-195

[73] Amato B, Coretti G, Compagna R, Amato M, Buffone G, Gigliotti D, et al. Role of matrix metalloproteinases in non-healing venous ulcers. International Wound Journal. 2015;**12**(6):641-645

[74] Gao M, Nguyen TT, Suckow MA, Wolter WR, Gooyit M, Mobashery S, et al. Acceleration of diabetic wound healing using a novel protease–anti-protease combination therapy. Proceedings of the National Academy of Sciences. 2015;**112**(49):15226-15231

[75] Nagase H, Woessner JF. Matrix metalloproteinases. Journal of Biological Chemistry. 1999;**274**(31):21491-21494

[76] Vu TH, Werb Z. Matrix metalloproteinases: Effectors of development and normal physiology. Genes & Development. 2000;**14**(17):2123-2133

[77] Lauer G, Sollberg S, Cole M, Krieg T, Eming SA, Flamme I, et al. Expression and proteolysis of vascular endothelial growth factor is increased in chronic wounds. Journal of Investigative Dermatology. 2000;**115**(1):12-18

[78] Krishnaswamy VR, Balaguru UM, Chatterjee S, Korrapati PS. Dermatopontin augments angiogenesis and modulates the expression of transforming growth factor beta 1 and integrin alpha 3 beta 1 in endothelial cells. European Journal of Cell Biology. 2017;**96**(3):266-275

[79] Serra R, Gallelli L, Grande R, Amato B, De Caridi G, Sammarco G, et al. Hemorrhoids and matrix metalloproteinases: A multicenter study on the predictive role of biomarkers. Surgery. 2016;**159**(2):487-494

[80] de Franciscis S, Mastroroberto P, Gallelli L, Buffone G, Montemurro R, Serra R. Increased plasma levels of metalloproteinase-9 and neutrophil gelatinase-associated lipocalin in a rare case of multiple artery aneurysm. Annals of Vascular Surgery. 2013;**27**(8):1185-e5

[81] Serra R, Buffone G, Falcone D, Molinari V, Scaramuzzino M, Gallelli L, et al. Chronic venous leg ulcers are associated with high levels of metalloproteinases-9 and neutrophil gelatinase-associated lipocalin. Wound Repair and Regeneration. 2013;**21**(3):395-401

[82] Abdollahi M, Ng TS, Rezaeizadeh A, Aamidor S, Twigg SM, Min D, et al. Insulin treatment prevents wounding associated changes in tissue and circulating neutrophil MMP-9 and NGAL in diabetic rats. PLoS One. 2017;**12**(2)

[83] Krampert M, Bloch W, Sasaki T, Bugnon P, Rulicke T, Wolf E, et al. Activities of the matrix metalloproteinase stromelysin-2 (MMP-10) in matrix degradation and keratinocyte organization in wounded skin. Molecular Biology of the Cell. 2004;**15**(12):5242-5254

[84] Bullard KM, Lund L, Mudgett JS, Mellin TN, Hunt TK, Murphy B, et al. Impaired wound contraction in stromelysin-1–deficient mice. Annals of Surgery. 1999;**230**(2):260

[85] Chen P, Abacherli LE, Nadler ST, Wang Y, Li Q, Parks WC. MMP7 shedding of syndecan-1 facilitates re-epithelialization by affecting α2β1 integrin activation. PLoS One. 2009;**4**(8)

[86] Mirastschijski U, Impola U, Jahkola T, Karlsmark T, Ågren MS, Saarialho-Kere U. Ectopic localization of matrix metalloproteinase-9 in chronic cutaneous wounds. Human Pathology. 2002;**33**(3):355-364

[87] Heng MC. Wound healing in adult skin: Aiming for perfect regeneration. International Journal of Dermatology. 2011;**50**(9):1058-1066

[88] Robson MC, Steed DL, Franz MG. Wound healing: Biologic features and approaches to maximize healing trajectories. Current Problems in Surgery. 2001;**2**(38):72-140

[89] Woo YC, Park SS, Subieta AR, Brennan TJ. Changes in tissue pH and temperature after incision indicate acidosis may contribute to postoperative pain. Anesthesiology: The Journal of the American Society of Anesthesiologists. 2004;**101**(2):468-475

[90] Werner S, Grose R. Regulation of wound healing by growth factors and cytokines. Physiological Reviews. 2003;**83**(3):835-870

[91] Heldin CH, Westermark B. Mechanism of action and in vivo role of platelet-derived growth factor. Physiological Reviews. 1999;**79**(4):1283-1316

[92] Park JH, Jeong YJ, Park KK, Cho HJ, Chung IK, Min KS, et al. Melittin suppresses PMA-induced tumor cell invasion by inhibiting NF-κB and AP-1-dependent MMP-9 expression. Molecules and Cells. 2010;**29**(2):209-215

[93] Momota Y, Suzuki N, Kasuya Y, Kobayashi T, Mizoguchi M, Yokoyama F, et al. Laminin alpha3 LG4 module induces keratinocyte migration involvement of matrix metalloproteinase-9. Journal of Receptor and Signal Transduction Research. 2005;**25**(1):1-17

[94] Giannelli G, Falk-Marzillier J, Schiraldi O, Stetler-Stevenson WG, Quaranta V. Induction of cell migration by matrix metalloprotease-2 cleavage of laminin-5. Science. 1997;**277**(5323):225-228

[95] Koshikawa N, Giannelli G, Cirulli V, Miyazaki K, Quaranta V. Role of cell surface metalloprotease MT1-MMP in epithelial cell migration over laminin-5. The Journal of Cell Biology. 2000;**148**(3):615-624

[96] Mäkelä M, Larjava H, Pirilä E, Maisi P, Salo T, Sorsa T, et al. Matrix metalloproteinase 2 (gelatinase A) is related to migration of keratinocytes. Experimental Cell Research. 1999;**251**(1):67-78

[97] McCawley LJ, O'Brien P, Hudson LG. Epidermal growth factor (EGF)-and scatter factor/hepatocyte growth factor (SF/HGF)-mediated keratinocyte migration is coincident with induction of matrix metalloproteinase (MMP)-9. Journal of Cellular Physiology. 1998;**176**(2):255-265

[98] da Cunha CB, Klumpers DD, Li WA, Koshy ST, Weaver JC, Chaudhuri O, et al. Influence of the stiffness of three-dimensional alginate/collagen-I interpenetrating networks on fibroblast biology. Biomaterials. 2014;**35**(32):8927-8936

[99] Jacinto A, Martinez-Arias A, Martin P. Mechanisms of epithelial fusion and repair. Nature Cell Biology. 2001;**3**(5):E117-E123

[100] Hinz B. Formation and function of the myofibroblast during tissue repair. Journal of Investigative Dermatology. 2007;**127**(3):526-537

[101] Wysocki AB, Staiano-Coico L, Grinneill F. Wound fluid from chronic leg ulcers contains elevated levels of metalloproteinases MMP-2 and MMP-9. Journal of Investigative Dermatology. 1993;**101**(1):64-68

[102] Takeo M, Lee W, Ito M. Wound healing and skin regeneration. Cold Spring Harbor Perspectives in Medicine. 2015;**5**(1):a023267

[103] Rosińczuk J, Taradaj J, Dymarek R, Sopel M. Mechanoregulation of wound healing and skin homeostasis. BioMed Research International. 2016;**2016**:3943481

[104] Arpino V, Brock M, Gill SE. The role of TIMPs in regulation of extracellular matrix proteolysis. Matrix Biology. 2015;**44**:247-254

[105] Sadowski T, Dietrich S, Müller M, Havlickova B, Schunck M, Proksch E, et al. Matrix metalloproteinase-19 expression in normal and diseased skin: Dysregulation by epidermal proliferation. Journal of Investigative Dermatology. 2003;**121**(5):989-996

[106] Inoue M, Kratz G, Haegerstrand A, Ståhle-Bäckdahl M. Collagenase expression is rapidly induced in wound-edge keratinocytes after acute injury in human skin, persists during healing, and stops at re-epithelialization. Journal of Investigative Dermatology. 1995;**104**(4):479-483

[107] Pilcher BK, Dumin JA, Sudbeck BD, Krane SM, Welgus HG, Parks WC. The activity of collagenase-1 is required for keratinocyte migration on a type I collagen matrix. The Journal of Cell Biology. 1997;**137**(6):1445-1457

[108] Di Colandrea T, Chada KK, Wang L, Wille J, D'Armiento J. Epidermal expression of collagenase delays wound-healing in transgenic mice. Journal of Investigative Dermatology. 1998;**111**(6):1029-1033

[109] Ravanti L, Toriseva M, Penttinen R, Crombleholme T, Foschi M, Han J, et al. Expression of human collagenase-3 (MMP-13) by fetal skin fibroblasts is induced by transforming growth factor β via p38 mitogen-activated protein kinase. The FASEB Journal. 2001;**15**(6):1098-1100

[110] Toriseva MJ, Ala-aho R, Karvinen J, Baker AH, Marjomäki VS, Heino J, et al. Collagenase-3 (MMP-13) enhances remodeling of three-dimensional collagen and promotes survival of human skin fibroblasts. Journal of Investigative Dermatology. 2007;**127**(1):49-59

[111] Holmbeck K, Bianco P, Caterina J, Yamada S, Kromer M, Kuznetsov SA, et al. MT1-MMP-deficient mice develop dwarfism, osteopenia, arthritis, and connective tissue disease due to inadequate collagen turnover. Cell. 1999;**99**(1):81-92

[112] Nissinen L, Kähäri VM. Matrix metalloproteinases in inflammation. Biochimica et Biophysica Acta (BBA) - General Subjects. 2014;**1840**(8):2571-2580

[113] Rechardt O, Vaalamo M, Höök-Nikanne J, Saarialho-Kere U, Elomaa O, Pääkkönen K, et al. Stromelysin-2 is upregulated during normal wound repair and is induced by cytokines. Journal of Investigative Dermatology. 2000;**115**(5):778-787

[114] Visse R, Nagase H. Matrix metalloproteinases and tissue inhibitors of metalloproteinases: Structure, function, and biochemistry. Circulation Research. 2003;**92**(8):827-839

[115] Chen W, Fu X, Ge S, Sun T, Sheng Z. Differential expression of matrix metalloproteinases and tissue-derived inhibitors of metalloproteinase in fetal and adult skins. International Journal of Biochemistry & Cell Biology. 2007;**39**(5):997-1005

[116] Mohan R, Chintala SK, Jung JC, Villar WV, McCabe F, Russo LA, et al. Matrix metalloproteinase gelatinase B (MMP-9) coordinates and effects epithelial regeneration. The Journal of Biological Chemistry. 2002;**277**(3):2065-2072

[117] Bergers G, Brekken R, McMahon G, Th V, Itoh T, Tamaki K, et al. Matrix metalloproteinase-9 triggers the angiogenic switch during carcinogenesis. Nature Cell Biology. 2000;**2**(10):737-744

[118] Chun TH, Sabeh F, Ota I, Murphy H, McDonagh KT, Holmbeck K, et al. MT1-MMP-dependent neovessel formation within the confines of the three-dimensional extracellular matrix. The Journal of Cell Biology. 2004;**167**(4):757-767

[119] Impola U, Toriseva M, Suomela S, Jeskanen L, Hieta N, Jahkola T, et al. Matrix metalloproteinase-19 is expressed by proliferating epithelium but disappears with neoplastic dedifferentiation. International Journal of Cancer. 2003;**103**(6):709-716

[120] Lazaro JL, Izzo V, Meaume S, Davies AH, Lobmann R, Uccioli L. Elevated levels of matrix metalloproteinases and chronic wound healing: An updated review of clinical evidence. Journal of Wound Care. 2016;**25**(5):277-287

[121] Rayment EA, Upton Z, Shooter GK. Increased matrix metalloproteinase-9 (MMP-9) activity observed in chronic wound fluid is related to the clinical severity of the ulcer. The British Journal of Dermatology. 2008;**158**(5):951-961

[122] Lobmann R, Ambrosch A, Schultz G, Waldmann K, Schiweck S, Lehnert H. Expression of matrix-metalloproteinases and their inhibitors in the wounds of diabetic and nondiabetic patients. Diabetologia. 2002;**45**(7):1011-1016

[123] Krisp C, Jacobsen F, McKay MJ, Molloy MP, Steinstraesser L, Wolters DA. Proteome analysis reveals antiangiogenic environments in chronic wounds of diabetes mellitus type 2 patients. Proteomics. 2013;**13**(17):2670-2681

[124] de Oliveira RR, Lemos A, de Castro Silveira PV, da Silva RJ, de Moraes SR. Alterations of tendons in patients with diabetes mellitus: A systematic review. Diabetic Medicine: A Journal of the British Diabetic Association. 2011;**28**(8):886-895

[125] Izzo V, Meloni M, Vainieri E, Giurato L, Ruotolo V, Uccioli L. High matrix metalloproteinase levels are associated with dermal graft failure in diabetic foot ulcers. The International Journal of Lower Extremity Wounds. 2014;**13**(3):191-196

[126] Kadoglou NP, Daskalopoulou SS, Perrea D, Liapis CD. Matrix metalloproteinases and diabetic vascular complications. Angiology. 2005;**56**(2):173-189

[127] Ban CR, Twigg SM. Fibrosis in diabetes complications: Pathogenic mechanisms and circulating and urinary markers. Vascular Health and Risk Management. 2008;**4**(3):575-596

[128] Mendias CL, Gumucio JP, Davis ME, Bromley CW, Davis CS, Brooks SV. Transforming growth factor-beta induces skeletal muscle atrophy and fibrosis through the induction of atrogin-1 and scleraxis. Muscle & Nerve. 2012;**45**(1):55-59

[129] Dinh T, Tecilazich F, Kafanas A, Doupis J, Gnardellis C, Leal E, et al. Mechanisms involved in the development and healing of diabetic foot ulceration. Diabetes. 2012;**61**(11):2937-2947

[130] Lu J, Guo JH, Xl T, Zhang C, Zhao M, Zhang QW, et al. Tiron inhibits UVB-induced AP-1 binding sites transcriptional activation on MMP-1 and MMP-3 promoters by MAPK signaling pathway in human dermal fibroblasts. PLoS One. 2016;**11**(8):e0159998

[131] Chung AW, Hsiang YN, Matzke LA, McManus BM, van Breemen C, Okon EB. Reduced expression of vascular endothelial growth factor paralleled with the increased angiostatin expression resulting from the upregulated activities of matrixmetalloproteinase-2 and -9 in human type 2 diabetic arterial vasculature. Circulation Research. 2006;**99**(2):140-148

[132] Death AK, Fisher EJ, McGrath KC, Yue DK. High glucose alters matrix metalloproteinase expression in two key vascular cells: Potential impact on atherosclerosis in diabetes. Atherosclerosis. 2003;**168**(2):263-269

[133] Yadav SS, Singh MK, Dwivedi P, Mandal RK, Usman K, Khattri S, et al. Significance of impaired serum gelatinases activities in metabolic syndrome. Toxicology International. 2014;**21**(1):107-111

[134] Li Z, Guo S, Yao F, Zhang Y, Li T. Increased ratio of serum matrix metalloproteinase-9 against TIMP-1 predicts poor wound healing in diabetic foot ulcers. Journal of Diabetes and its Complications. 2013;**27**(4):380-382

[135] Menghini R, Uccioli L, Vainieri E, Pecchioli C, Casagrande V, Stoehr R, et al. Expression of tissue inhibitor of metalloprotease 3 is reduced in ischemic but not neuropathic ulcers from patients with type 2 diabetes mellitus. Acta Diabetologica. 2013;**50**(6):907-910

[136] Lopez-Lopez N, Gonzalez-Curiel I, Trevino-Santa Cruz MB, Rivas-Santiago B, TrujilloPaez V, Enciso-Moreno JA, et al. Expression and vitamin D-mediated regulation of matrix metalloproteinases (MMPs) and tissue inhibitors of metalloproteinases (TIMPs) in healthy skin and in diabetic foot ulcers. Archives of Dermatological Research. 2014;**306**(9):809-821

[137] Burrow JW, Koch JA, Chuang HH, Zhong W, Dean DD, Sylvia VL. Nitric oxide donors selectively reduce the expression of matrix metalloproteinases-8 and -9 by human diabetic skin fibroblasts. The Journal of Surgical Research. 2007;**140**(1):90-98

[138] Overall CM, Kleifeld O. Towards third generation matrix

metalloproteinase inhibitors for cancer therapy. British Journal of Cancer. 2006;**94**(7):941-946

[139] Amar S, Minond D, Fields GB. Clinical implications of compounds designed to inhibit ECM-modifying metalloproteinases. Proteomics. 2017;**17**(23-24):1600389

[140] Gooyit M, Peng Z, Wolter WR, Pi H, Ding D, Hesek D, et al. A chemical biological strategy to facilitate diabetic wound healing. ACS Chemical Biology. 2014;**9**(1):105-110

[141] Nguyen TT, Ding D, Wolter WR, Pérez RL, Champion MM, Mahasenan KV, et al. Validation of matrix metalloproteinase-9 (MMP-9) as a novel target for treatment of diabetic foot ulcers in humans and discovery of a potent and selective small-molecule MMP-9 inhibitor that accelerates healing. Journal of Medicinal Chemistry. 2018;**61**(19):8825-8837

[142] Appleby TC, Greenstein AE, Hung M, Liclican A, Velasquez M, Villaseñor AG, et al. Biochemical characterization and structure determination of a potent, selective antibody inhibitor of human MMP9. Journal of Biological Chemistry. 2017;**292**(16):6810-6820

[143] Bendell JC, Starodub A, Shah MA, Sharma S, Wainberg ZA, Thai DL. Phase I study of GS-5745 alone and in combination with chemotherapy in patients with advanced solid tumors. Journal of Clinical Oncology. 2015;**33**(Suppl 15):4030-4030

[144] Shah MA, Starodub A, Sharma S, Berlin J, Patel M, Wainberg ZA, et al. Andecaliximab/GS-5745 alone and combined with mFOLFOX6 in advanced gastric and gastroesophageal junction adenocarcinoma: Results from a phase I study. Clinical Cancer Research. 2018;**24**(16):3829-3837

[145] Sela-Passwell N, Kikkeri R, Dym O, Rozenberg H, Margalit R, Arad-Yellin R, et al. Antibodies targeting the catalytic zinc complex of activated matrix metalloproteinases show therapeutic potential. Nature Medicine. 2012;**18**(1):143

[146] Hu J, Van den Steen PE, Houde M, Ilenchuk TT, Opdenakker G. Inhibitors of gelatinase B/matrix metalloproteinase-9 activity: Comparison of a peptidomimetic and polyhistidine with single-chain derivatives of a neutralizing monoclonal antibody. Biochemical Pharmacology. 2004;**67**(5):1001-1009

[147] Paemen L, Martens E, Masure S, Opdenakker G. Monoclonal antibodies specific for natural human neutrophil gelatinase B used for affinity purification, quantitation by two-site ELISA and inhibition of enzymatic activity. European Journal of Biochemistry. 1995;**234**(3):759-765

[148] Hariono M, Yuliani SH, Istyastono EP, Riswanto FD, AdhipanditoCF.Matrixmetalloproteinase 9 (MMP9) in wound healing of diabetic foot ulcer: Molecular target and structure-based drug design. Wound Medicine. 2018;**22**:1-3

[149] Vowden K, Vowden P. Wound dressings: Principles and practice. Surgery. 2014;**32**:462-467

[150] Rayment EA, Dargaville TR, Shooter GK, George GA, Upton Z. Attenuation of protease activity in chronic wound fluid with bisphosphonate-functionalised hydrogels. Biomaterials. 2008;**29**(12):1785-1795

[151] Tronci G, Yin J, Holmes RA, Liang H, Russell SJ, Wood DJ. Protease-sensitive atelocollagen hydrogels promote healing in a diabetic wound model. Journal of Materials Chemistry B. 2016;**4**(45):7249-7258

[152] Ågren MS, Mirastschijski U, Karlsmark T, Saarialho-Kere UK. Topical synthetic inhibitor of matrix metalloproteinases delays epidermal regeneration of human wounds. Experimental Dermatology. 2001;**10**(5):337-348

[153] Jeong EH, Kim H, Jang B, Cho H, Ryu J, Kim B, et al. Technological development of structural DNA/RNA-based RNAi systems and their applications. Advanced Drug Delivery Reviews. 2016;**104**:29-43

[154] Wang J, Lu Z, Wientjes MG, Au JL. Delivery of siRNA therapeutics: Barriers and carriers. The AAPS Journal. 2010;**12**(4):492-503

[155] Georgiou TK, Vamvakaki M, Patrickios CS, Yamasaki EN, Phylactou LA. Nanoscopic cationic methacrylate star homopolymers: Synthesis by group transfer polymerization, characterization and evaluation as transfection reagents. Biomacromolecules. 2004;**5**(6):2221-2229

[156] Srinivasachari S, Fichter KM, Reineke TM. Polycationic β-cyclodextrin "click clusters": Monodisperse and versatile scaffolds for nucleic acid delivery. Journal of the American Chemical Society. 2008;**130**(14):4618-4627

[157] Xu FJ, Zhang ZX, Ping Y, Li J, Kang ET, Neoh KG. Star-shaped cationic polymers by atom transfer radical polymerization from β-cyclodextrin cores for nonviral gene delivery. Biomacromolecules. 2009;**10**(2):285-293

[158] Cryan SA, Holohan A, Donohue R, Darcy R, O'Driscoll CM. Cell transfection with polycationic cyclodextrin vectors. European Journal of Pharmaceutical Sciences. 2004;**21**(5):625-633

[159] Yang C, Zhu P, Yan L, Chen L, Meng R, Lao G. Dynamic changes in matrix metalloproteinase 9 and tissue inhibitor of metalloproteinase 1 levels during wound healing in diabetic rats. Journal of the American Podiatric Medical Association. 2009;**99**(6):489-496

[160] Li N, Luo HC, Yang C, Deng JJ, Ren M, Xie XY, et al. Cationic star-shaped polymer as an siRNA carrier for reducing MMP-9 expression in skin fibroblast cells and promoting wound healing in diabetic rats. International Journal of Nanomedicine. 2014;**9**:3377

[161] Li N, Luo HC, Ren M, Zhang LM, Wang W, Pan CL, et al. Efficiency and safety of β-CD-(D3) 7 as siRNA carrier for decreasing matrix metalloproteinase-9 expression and improving wound healing in diabetic rats. ACS Applied Materials & Interfaces. 2017;**9**(20):17417-17426

[162] Wang W, Yang C, Yi Wang X, Yan Zhou L, Juan Lao G, Liu D, et al. MicroRNA-129 and-335 promote diabetic wound healing by inhibiting Sp1-mediated MMP-9 expression. Diabetes. 2018;**67**(8):1627-1638

[163] Rah B, Amin H, Yousuf K, Khan S, Jamwal G, Mukherjee D, et al. A novel MMP-2 inhibitor 3-azidowithaferin A (3-azidoWA) abrogates cancer cell invasion and angiogenesis by modulating extracellular Par-4. PLoS One. 2012;7(9):e44039

[164] Ji BC, Hsiao YP, Tsai CH, Chang SJ, Hsu SC, Liu HC, et al. Cantharidin impairs cell migration and invasion of A375. S2 human melanoma cells by suppressing MMP-2 and-9 through PI3K/NF-κB signaling pathways. Anticancer Research. 2015;**35**(2):729-738

[165] Wang Z, Zhai Z, Du X. Celastrol inhibits migration and invasion

through blocking the NF-κB pathway in ovarian cancer cells. Experimental and Therapeutic Medicine. 2017; **14**(1):819-824

[166] Liu KC, Huang AC, Wu PP, Lin HY, Chueh FS, Yang JS, et al. Gallic acid suppresses the migration and invasion of PC-3 human prostate cancer cells via inhibition of matrix metalloproteinase-2 and-9 signaling pathways. Oncology Reports. 2011;**26**(1):177-184

[167] Kim WK, Song SY, Oh WK, Kaewsuwan S, Tran TL, Kim WS, et al. Wound-healing effect of ginsenoside Rd from leaves of *Panax ginseng* via cyclic AMP-dependent protein kinase pathway. European Journal of Pharmacology. 2013;**702**(1-3):285-293

[168] Liu W, Zhang Q, Tang Q, Hu C, Huang J, Liu Y, et al. Lycorine inhibits cell proliferation and migration by inhibiting ROCK1/cofilin-induced actin dynamics in HepG2 hepatoblastoma cells. Oncology Reports. 2018;**40**(4):2298-2306

[169] Aroui S, Aouey B, Chtourou Y, Meunier AC, Fetoui H, Kenani A. Naringin suppresses cell metastasis and the expression of matrix metalloproteinases (MMP-2 and MMP-9) via the inhibition of ERK-P38-JNK signaling pathway in human glioblastoma. Chemico-Biological Interactions. 2016;**244**:195-203

[170] Park EJ, Park HJ, Chung HJ, Shin Y, Min HY, Hong JY, et al. Antimetastatic activity of pinosylvin, a natural stilbenoid, is associated with the suppression of matrix metalloproteinases. The Journal of Nutritional Biochemistry. 2012;**23**(8):946-952

[171] Chun J, Kim YS. Platycodin D inhibits migration, invasion, and growth of MDA-MB-231 human breast cancer cells via suppression of EGFR-mediated Akt and MAPK pathways. Chemico-Biological Interactions. 2013;**205**(3):212-221

[172] Zhou R, Xu L, Ye M, Liao M, Du H, Chen H. Formononetin inhibits migration and invasion of MDA-MB-231 and 4T1 breast cancer cells by suppressing MMP-2 and MMP-9 through PI3K/AKT signaling pathways. Hormone and Metabolic Research. 2014;**46**(11):753-760

[173] Zeng S, Zhu B, Zeng J, Wu W, Jiang C. Zeylenone represses the progress of human prostate cancer by downregulating the Wnt/β-catenin pathway. Molecular Medicine Reports. 2018;**18**(6):5572-5578

[174] Yen YH, Pu CM, Liu CW, Chen YC, Chen YC, Liang CJ, et al. Curcumin accelerates cutaneous wound healing via multiple biological actions: The involvement of TNF-α, MMP-9, α-SMA, and collagen. International Wound Journal. 2018;**15**(4):605-617

[175] Deng B, Qiu B. Shikonin inhibits invasiveness of osteosarcoma through MMP13 suppression. Tumor Biology. 2015;**36**(12):9311-9317

[176] Zhang FY, Hu Y, Que ZY, Wang P, Liu YH, Wang ZH, et al. Shikonin inhibits the migration and invasion of human glioblastoma cells by targeting phosphorylated β-catenin and phosphorylated PI3K/Akt: A potential mechanism for the anti-glioma efficacy of a traditional Chinese herbal medicine. International Journal of Molecular Sciences. 2015;**16**(10):23823-23848

Chapter 6

Novel Application of Immunomodulatory Mushroom Polysaccharide (β-Glucan) and Triterpenes for Diabetic Wound Care

Shiu-Nan Chen, Yu-Sheng Wu, Sherwin Chen,
Ya-Chin Chang and Chung-Lun Lu

Abstract

β-Glucan and triterpenes are two important derivative compounds from traditional medicinal mushroom, such as *Ganoderma lucidum* and *Antrodia cinnamomea*. β-glucan and triterpenes are considered to have immunoregulatory properties in disease treatment for long years. The immunoregulatory effects are usually activated through some transcription of pro-inflammatory genes and possess immunomodulatory activity. Difficulty in healing wound now is a common condition that occurred in diabetic patients, and the physiological hyperglycemic status of diabetic patients resulting in the wounds continue to produce an inflammatory response. Thus, we hope to use β-glucan and triterpenes for difficult wound healing that possess immunomodulatory activity on the wound micro-environment and stimulate the positive effects on healing. In this chapter, these two important derivative compounds from traditional medicinal mushroom were examined by diabetic mammal's wound healing models. In these models, the skin wounds' microenvironment is expected close to diabetic foot, suffering in hyperglycemic and inflammatory status. The results are clearly presented, with the immunomodulatory effects from mushroom β-glucan and triterpenes that involved in modulating the cell-mediated immune system to cause cellular proliferation and further to introduce healing performance of the chronic inflammation wounds.

Keywords: mushroom polysaccharide, β-glucans, triterpenes, immunomodulatory, diabetic, wound healing

1. Introduction

Diabetes is a metabolic disease characterized by hyperglycemia resulting from defects in insulin secretion or function, and is associated with the long-term damage, dysfunction, and failure of various organs, especially the eyes, kidneys, nerves, heart, and blood vessels [1]. One of the main consequences of diabetes is the impairment of self-repairing abilities [2]. Various studies have indicated that diets high in saturated fat and cholesterol contribute to hypercholesterolemia and metabolic disturbances, which may cause hyperglycemic condition in humans and animals [3]. Hyperglycemia can rapidly become severe hyperglycemia and/or ketoacidosis in the presence of infection or other types of stress. The inducing stress can result from the presence of excessive counter regulatory hormones (glucagon, growth hormone, catecholamine, and glucocorticoid; either endogenous or exogenous) and high circulating or tissue levels of inflammatory cytokine [1, 4]. As many reports have shown, a wound healing is an intricate regulation mechanism, which involves many cell populations and molecular mediators, and is one of the key mechanisms that ensures the barrier functions of the skin and the maintenance of body homeostasis. The efficiency of this process is largely determined by the balance of proinflammatory and proregenerative signals, which are mediated by cytokines [5, 6]. But in patients who suffer from diabetes mellitus, chronic wounds occur often due to the impairment of wound healing; major complications of diabetes lead to inflammation and oxidative stress, delayed wound healing, and persistent ulcers. The impaired healing in diabetes is the result of a complex pathophysiology involving vascular, neuropathic, immune, and biochemical components. Hyperglycemia correlates with stiffer blood vessels, which cause slower circulation and microvascular dysfunction, causing reduced tissue oxygenation. Blood vessel alterations observed in diabetic patients also account for reduced leukocyte migration into the wound, which becomes more vulnerable to infections. The hyperglycemic environment itself can compromise leucocyte function. In addition, peripheral neuropathy can lead to numbness of the area and reduced ability to feel pain, which can lead to chronicization of wounds that are not immediately noticed and properly treated [7].

In this chapter, two immunomodulatory extracts (β-glucan and triterpenes) from popular medicinal mushroom were assessed by scientific experiments to examine the functions for treating poorly healing wounds. These immunomodulatory extracts have been studied for its biological effects in mammals widely, and reported to possess antitumor and immunomodulating activities with anti-inflammatory effects and the ability to control tissue cytokines [8–10]. Here, the scientific experiment results of wound healing were consolidated and the novel application of derivative compounds from traditional medicinal mushroom can be used for treatment of diabetic foot in the future.

2. β-Glucan from mushroom and its diabetic wound caring

2.1 Mushroom β-glucan functions for wound caring

Glucan is a polysaccharide structure which is constructed by D-glucose, linked by glycosidic bonds. It is now a common product usually obtained by extracting its components from fungi [11] (such as mushrooms) or yeast cell walls and it has been known in recent studies to effectively stimulate immune cells; it not only can enhance specific immune responses of the organism, but also enhance the nonspecific immune response, and is a good immune regulator. One group of the glucan, the beta-glucans (β-glucans), is a heterogeneous group of glucose polymers consisting of β-(1,3)-linked β-d-glucopyranosyl units with a β-(1,6)-linked side chain of varying distribution and lengths. These polysaccharides are of different chemical compositions, with most belonging to the group of β-glucans; these have β-(1 → 3) linkages in the primary chain of the glucan and additional β-(1 → 6) branch points that are needed for their bioactive response [12, 13]. Many species of mushroom can produce glucan, such as *Ganoderma lucidum, Grifola frondosa, Pleurotus ostreatus, Lentinula edodes, Cordyceps militaris*, and so on [14].

Research on β-glucans application has indicated that this bioactive immunomodulating substance not only enhances the organism's ability to resist infection by bacteria, fungi, viruses, and parasites, but even has the effect of inhibiting tumor growth [15]. This novel immunomodulating substance is thought to mediate effects through activation of various immune system components including macrophages, neutrophils, natural killer (NK) cells, and lymphocytes. Moreover, they are demonstrated to possess immunostimulatory activity and enhance wound healing especially by increasing macrophage infiltration into the injury sites and stimulating tissue regeneration [16].

In the field of wound healing, it has been pointed out by many related studies that by activating macrophages, β-glucan can stimulate the regeneration of collagen and help wound healing [17]. In 2001, Kougias and others found that in addition to the receptors on immune cells, (1-3)-β-D-glucans receptors were also found on human dermal fibroblasts. Making fibroblasts directly receive messages from glucans represents a factor that promotes wound healing not only by activating macrophages, but also by stimulating fibroblasts [18]. In study of the mechanism between fibroblasts and wound healing, we can find that after being stimulated by β-glucan, fibroblasts activate two translation factors (transcription factors)-AP-1 (activator protein-1), SP1 (specific protein-1), and two signaling pathways-NF-κB (nuclear factor-κB), NF-1 (nuclear factor-1), can strengthen the immune response at the wound site and promote the hyperplasia and the expression of collagen precursor genes (procollagen genes), thereby generating collagen, to achieve the effect of wound healing [18, 19]. The results from a reference illustrated that mushroom polysaccharides derived from Schizophyllum (1-3),(1-6)-β-D-glucans, were mixed with gelatin to make artificial skin, either by in vitro cell culture or transplanted into mice, which led to the observation of the growth of new tissues and finding that they all have the effect of promoting epidermal cellization [20]. Mushroom β-glucan's (MBG) role has also been confirmed in tests on the recovery of liver cuts in fish and skin wounds in rats. By stimulating the mechanism of Wnt/β catenin signaling signal transmission, liver cell hyperplasia, and cellular activity, it promotes wound healing [13]. In the application of β-D-glucans in wound healing, it has a reduced chance of infection after surgery [21]; the synthesis of polysaccharides and collagen matrix can promote the recovery of local deep scald skin also has a medical effect for the relief of patients' pain [22].

2.2 Mushroom β-glucan (MBG) applied in advanced dressing to promote diabetic wound healing (mammal testing model)

In 2018, we carried out a study on mushroom β-glucan (MBG) from *G. lucidum* for testing wound healing in animals. The purified β-glucan of *G. lucidum* was mixed with carboxymethyl cellulose fiber and water, and then through Poly-charge/ion exchange for compounding, and the composite fiber solution is prepared into a fiber sponge substrate by a freeze-drying process, that patented technology from Taiwan Textile Research Institute, to form a sponge dressing contain mushroom β-glucan (**Figure 1(a)**). Carboxymethyl cellulose fibers and β-glucan form the structure of a sponge, and the mushroom β-glucan-containing particles are evenly dispersed in the fiber sponge (**Figure 1(b)**). The swelling ratio of the fiber sponge substrate sample is about 22–32 times. It has the effect of absorbing fluid, which means that it can provide the effect of absorbing too much exudate if it is used on wounds with a lot of exudate, and maintain the proper moisture of the wound to promote wound healing.

The prepared fiber sponge substrate has a high magnification of moisture absorption and swelling ratio and an appropriate structural stability that causes the

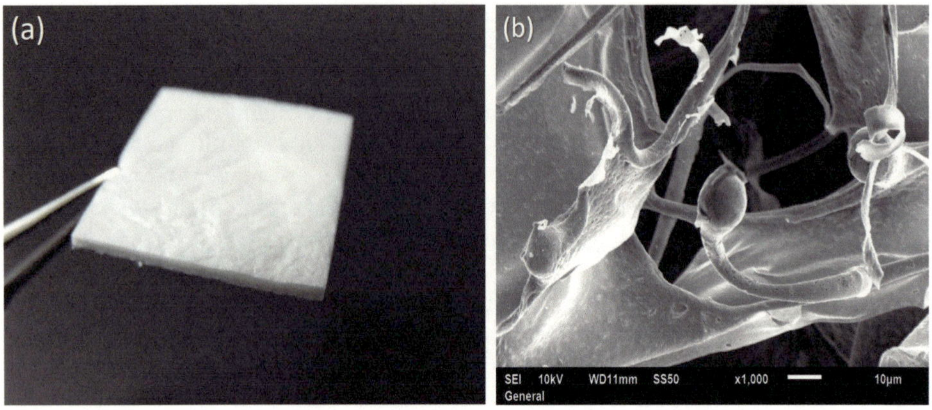

Figure 1.
Mushroom β-glucan-containing bio-fiber sponge dressing. (a) Appearance of mushroom β-glucan-containing bio-fiber sponge dressing; (b) mushroom β-glucan-containing particles dispersed in the fiber sponge structure (1000×).

release of mushroom β-glucan (MBG) in the substrate slowly. It is expected that it will have an extended-release ability to produce immunostimulatory polysaccharides, which can improve the shortcomings of commercially available sponge dressing products.

In an experiment using three diabetic model pigs, we explored whether mushroom β-glucan (MBG) sponge dressing can accelerate wound healing rate when applied to man-cut wounds. For the present study, all the mammal experiments were performed in accordance with protocol by the Institutional Animal Care and Use Committee (IACUC) of Agricultural Technology Research Institute (ATRI, in Taiwan). Type I diabetes pigs were manual Streptozotocin-induced (to generate chronic wound healing), housed, and surgery was operated in SPF animal room facilities by ATRI Animal Technology Laboratories. Six square wounds (2 ± 0.5 cm × 2 ± 0.5 cm) with full skin layer on the back of one pig were formed by manual operation, three on each side, L1, L2, L3 on the left;R1, R2, R3 on the right (schematic diagram in **Figure 2**), and randomly apply the test mushroom β-glucan (MBG) sponge dressing or control dressing to the wound in the above. Then, the wound healing of each test substance was continuously observed, and the effect of the test substance

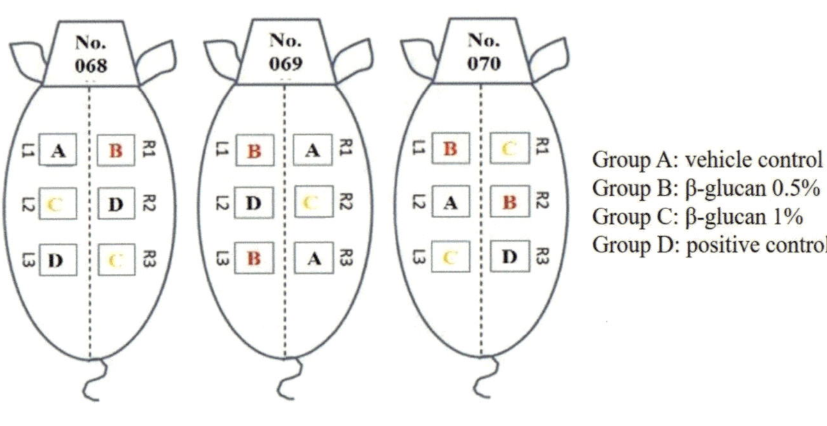

Figure 2.
Wounds with full skin layer on the diabetic pig. Six square wounds (2 ± 0.5 cm × 2 ± 0.5 cm) with full skin layer on pigs were formed by manual operation, randomly apply the test mushroom β-glucan (MBG) sponge dressing or control dressing to the wound in the above (three pigs, each test dressing N = 4 or 5).

on wound healing was explored based on pathological interpretation. During the test period, the test substances in each group did not affect the growth of the pigs and also did not cause death.

In data calculation, the average value (mean) and standard error of the mean (SEM) of each test group were calculated by Microsoft Excel, and finally presented in the report as mean ± SEM. In statistical analysis, one-way ANOVA was performed with IBM SPSS Statistics 20 analysis software, and the Scheffe's post-mortem analysis method was used. The lowercase letter labels in figures mean that there is a significant difference between those who do not have the same letter at the observation time point ($p < 0.05$). In the experimental results, on the 10th day of the experiment, the secretion of tissue fluid of each test group decreased, and it was observed that the granulation tissue had grown to fill the entire wound, forming a bright red and smooth appearance, and the neonatal epithelial tissue could be observed at the edge of the wound, the wound area was significantly reduced, for example in **Figure 3**. The degree of wound healing speed was group B: 51.1% > group D: 49.2% > group C: 44.3% > group A: 41.0%. In statistical analysis results: group A and group B, group A and group C, group A and group D reach statistical significance $p < 0.05$. The statistical significance of group B and C was not more than $p > 0.05$, and the statistical significance of group B and D was not more than $p > 0.05$. Group C and D did not reach statistical significance $p > 0.05$. The test mushroom β-glucan (MBG) sponge dressing showed better wound healing performance than vehicle control (**Figure 4**).

In the histopathological examination result, the thickness of the skin dermal layer and epidermal layer were measured to evaluate the wound healing. In the

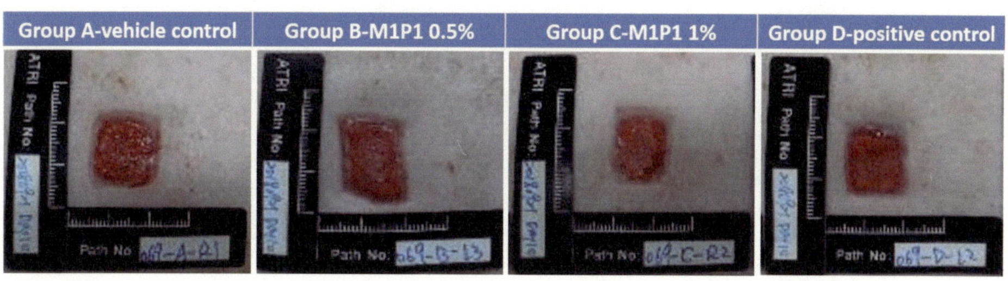

Figure 3.
Ten days' observation result at the edge of the wound. The performance of wound healing appearance at 10th day, the granulation tissue had grown to fill the entire wound, forming a bright red and smooth appearance, and the neonatal epithelial tissue could be observed at the edge of the wound.

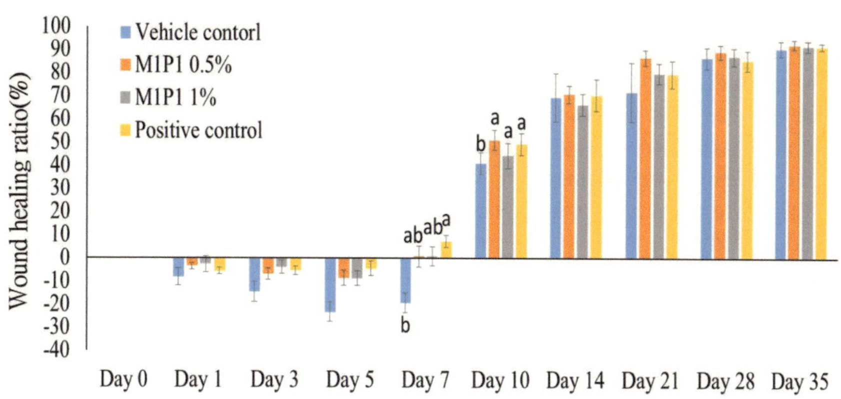

Figure 4.
Wound healing ratio.

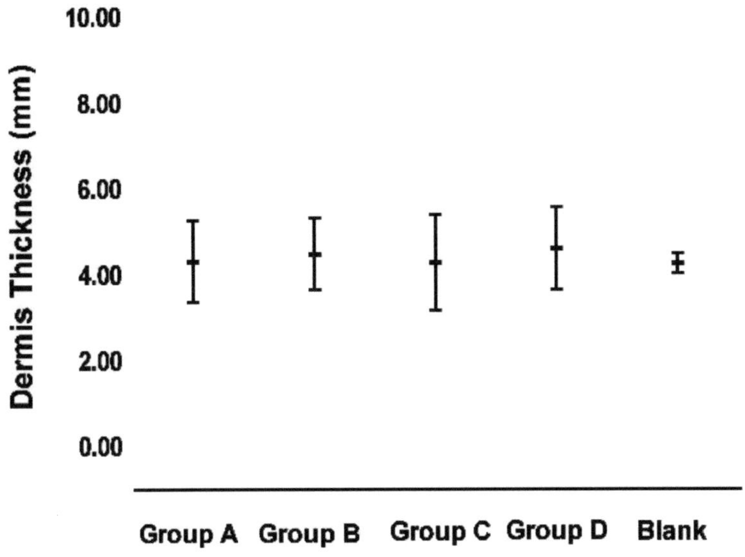

Figure 5.
The thickness of the skin dermal layer of the animals in each test group.

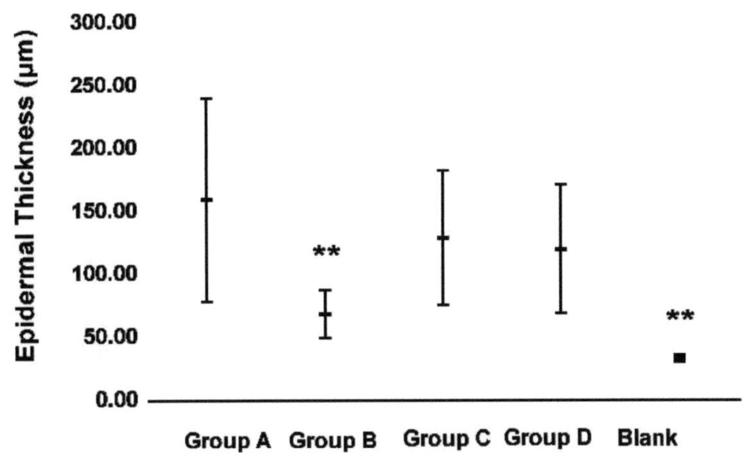

Figure 6.
The thickness of the epidermal layer of the animals in each test group.

diabetic pig model, the thickness of the skin dermal layer of the animals in each test group was not different from each other (**Figure 5**). The analysis of the thickness of the epidermal layer showed that the thickness of the test group A is significantly higher than that of mushroom β-glucan (MBG) sponge dressing (test group B) ($p < 0.01$) (**Figure 6**). Epidermal cell layer tissue formation (epithelization) showed that the wound healing of each group of animals in the diabetic pig model was good, and there was no statistical difference between the test groups in the evaluation of epithelial cell formation response (**Figure 7**).

The results of wound healing tissue react evaluation showed that the inflammatory reaction of animal skin in test group B and test group D was significantly higher than that in control group (test group A) with statistical difference ($p < 0.01$). In addition, the degree of inflammatory response stimulation in test group C was significantly slowed down compared with the positive control group (test group D), indicating that test group B and test group D stimulated local skin inflammation and

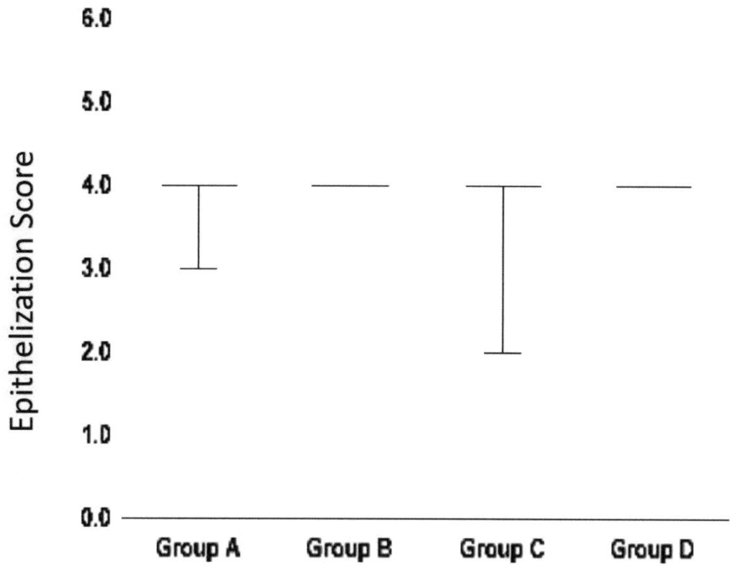

Figure 7.
The evaluation of epithelial cell formation response of the animals in each test group.

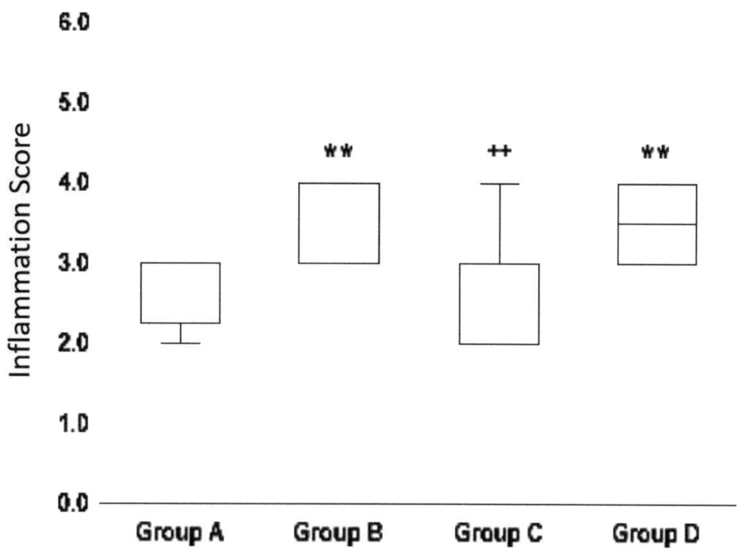

Figure 8.
The degree of inflammatory response stimulation of the animals in each test group.

accelerated skin wound healing, but significantly slowed down in the experimental group C (**Figure 8**). After assay of the degree of skin blood capillary, the experimental group B (M1P1 0.5%) can be observed that the response is statistically different from the control group (test group A), showing that the new blood capillary of test substance is more effective than the control group (test group A) in wound healing (**Figure 9**). Moreover, section slices of recovered wound indicated that mushroom β-glucan (MBG) sponge dressing treatment revealed better wound tissue flatness effects than untreated group and positive control (**Figure 10(a)-(d)**).

In conclusion, based on the results of epidermal layer, dermal layer thickness and the local tissue reaction of wound healing, the mushroom β-glucan (MBG) sponge dressing M1P1 0.5% treatment group (test group B) is more effective in wound

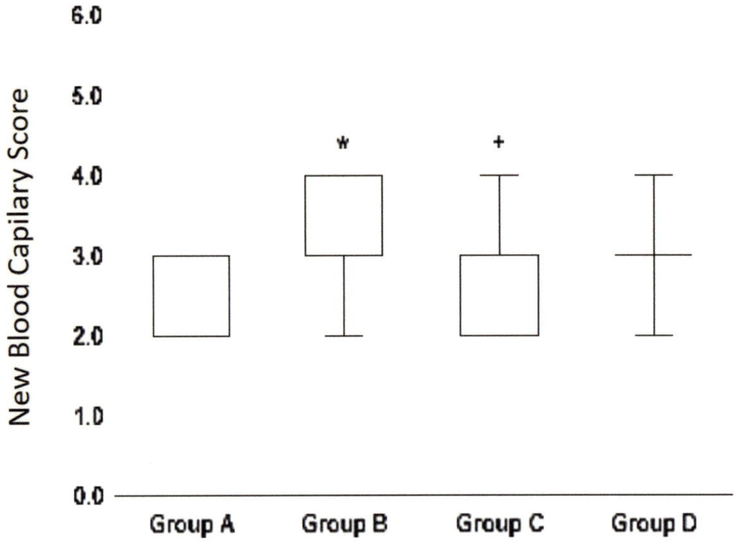

Figure 9.
The degree of skin new blood capillary in each test group.

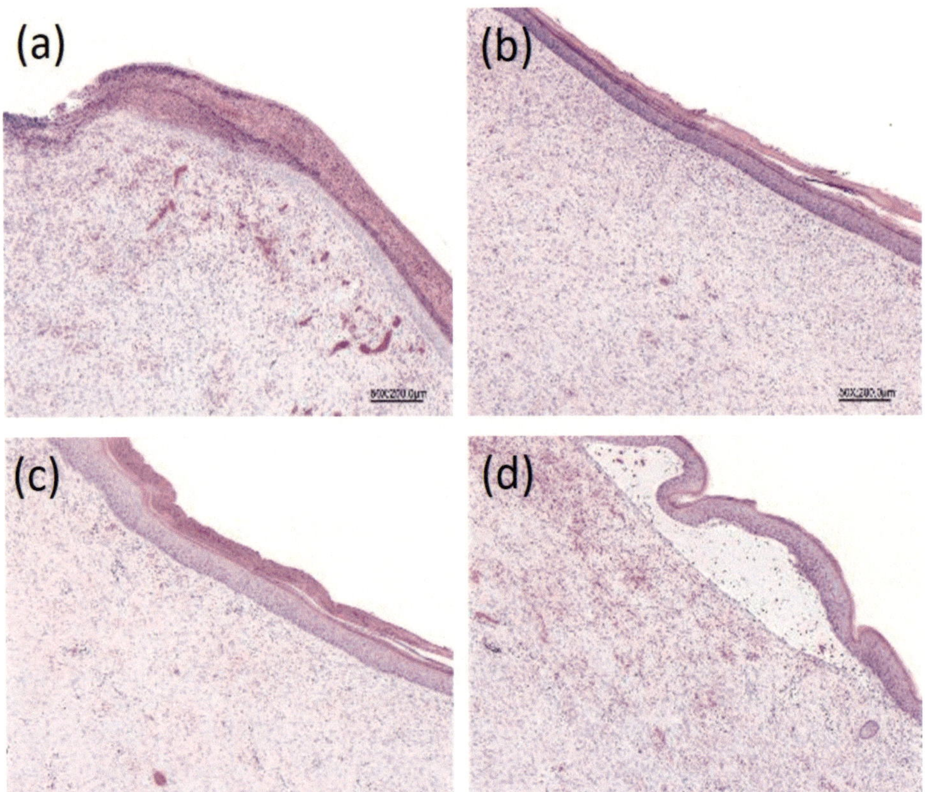

Figure 10.
Section slices of recovered wound in each test group. (a) Animal ID: 068-L1 H&E staining, 50×. Group A; (b) animal ID: 069-L3 H&E staining, 50×. Group B; (c) animal ID: 070-R1 H&E staining, 50×. Group C; (d) animal ID: 069-L2 H&E staining, 50×. Group D. Mushroom β-glucan (MBG) sponge dressing treatment (b and c) reveals better wound tissue flatness effects than untreated group and positive control.

healing than the test substance treatment group C (M1P1 1%) and the positive control group (test group D). When the mushroom β-glucan was applied on diabetic pigs wound, we expected the bioactive immunomodulation from mushroom β-glucan (MBG) occurred in chronic wound microenvironment, and promote wound healing.

3. Triterpenes from *Antrodia cinnamomea* in wound caring

3.1 *Antrodia cinnamomea* triterpenes for wound caring

Since antiquity, mushrooms have been valued by humankind as a culinary wonder and folk medicine in Oriental practice. In recent years, mushrooms have emerged as a source of dietary supplements, antioxidants, anticancer, prebiotic, immunomodulating, anti-inflammatory, cardiovascular, antimicrobial, and antidiabetic functions [23]. Among the different types of mushrooms, *A. cinnamomea* is a special fungal parasite that grows on the inner cavity of the endemic species of *Cinnamomum kanehirae* (Bull camphor tree) in Taiwan [24]. This mushroom is considered as a highly valued mushroom due to its rare occurrence, cultivation difficulties of fruit bodies and its common uses as a traditional herb for the treatment of several ailments such as diarrhea, abdominal pain, hypertension, itchy skin, etc. [24, 25]. In Asia, *A. cinnamomea* dried mycelia powder is officially recognized as a rare dietary supplement. Given its popularity, in recent years, fermentation techniques have been employed in the mass production of *A. cinnamomea* and its products have been marketed as functional foods for over 10 years. Among the several bioactive or functional compounds such as polysaccharides, polysaccharides-peptides, nucleosides, and triterpenes that are reported to possess therapeutic effects from *A. cinnamomea*, bioactive *A. cinnamomea* triterpenes were reported with the activity to possess antitumor and immunomodulating activities with anti-inflammatory effects [8], and apoptotic effects in the leukemia HL-60 cells, which suggest that the triterpenes extract may possess protective antioxidants and anticancer properties for biophysiology [26].

Several plant derivatives, such as secondary metabolites, are capable of promoting wound healing in various animal models. A group of secondary metabolites attracting much attention is the pentacyclic triterpenes [27, 28]. Triterpenes, a large and structurally diverse group of natural products derived from squalene or related acyclic 30-carbon precursors, are uniquely abundant with well-characterized biological activities of modulation on the immune cells [29]. In surgical wounds, the triterpenes induced a reduction in time to closure, and this effect was reported in virtually all wound types. In references, triterpenes also modulate the production of ROS in the wound microenvironment, accelerating the process of tissue repair through inducing cell migration, cell proliferation, and collagen deposition [27].

According to these findings and hypotheses, we used triterpenes extracted from *A. cinnamomea* mycelium to examine anti-inflammatory responses in STZ-induced hyperglycemic mice by oral treatment and observed the effect of triterpenes on wound healing model in the mice, and the complete results were published in paper in 2016 [30].

3.2 *Antrodia cinnamomea* triterpenes promote wound healing in hyperglycemic diabetic mice model

The *A. cinnamomea* BCRC36401 was purchased from the Bioresources Collection and Research Center (BCRC), Food Industry Research and Development

Institute, Hsinchu, Taiwan. In laboratory culture system, the *A. cinnamomea* was subcultured into oats containing 5% glucose (16301, RDH) and 1% yeast extract (09182, SIGMA) within the vent plug-glass bottles at 22°C with 12 h of light for 30 days. After the mycelium was observed to overlap on the cultured oats, the mycelia were separated from fermented broth and washed with distilled water. Finally, the mycelia were freeze-dried to powders. The freeze-dried powder was initiated into the 80°C hot water for 6 h (powder:hot water = 1:100) to separate the water-soluble materials. After removal of water-soluble materials, the extraction of triterpenes was performed using 99.8% water-free ethanol (SIGMA) (the removed water-soluble powder:water-free ethanol = 1:50) in 1.5 h three times, and then lyophilized. The extracted compound was used in testing and analysis of triterpenes species by HPLC (**Figure 11**). The *A. cinnamomea* extract analyzed by HPLC was compared to the 11 species of triterpenes and the results was indicated that it was including of Antcin H, Dehydrosulphurenic acid, Eburicoic acid, Methyl antcinate B and Dehydroeburicoic acid (**Table 1**). The recovery rate was measured from different weight of the powder and the presented recovery rate about 7–10%.

Diabetes mouse skin wound healing examination was carried out following the wound healing model assay procedure [13, 31]. All study procedures were performed in accordance with protocol approved by the National Taiwan University Animal and Use Committee (NTUAUC). We used 15 of 6-week-old male ICR (N = 3, purchased from Laboratory Animal Center, National Taiwan University College of Medicine) for this experiment, and animals were housed in the Animal Housing Facility of National Taiwan University, College of Life Science. At the beginning, manual incision wound (one of $1.5 \times 0.5\ cm^2$ full thickness) was made on mice skin. Each wound was cleaned by the 3 M Cavilon™ No Rinse-Skin

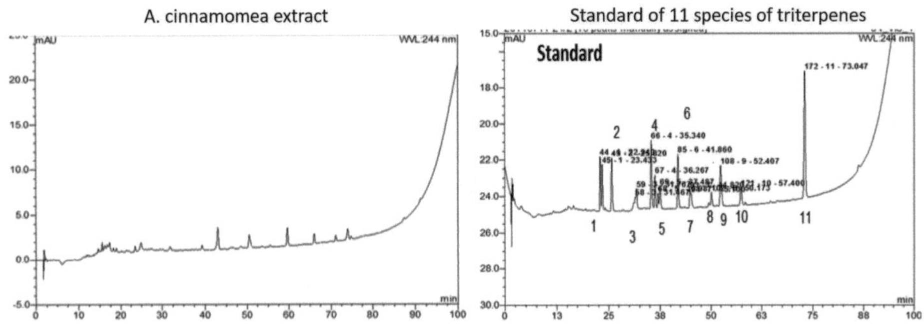

Figure 11.
HPLC identification of A. cinnamomea *extracted triterpenes. (Left) HPLC result of* A. cinnamomea *extract; (right) standard of the 11 species of triterpenes.*

Retention time	Predicted triterpenes species	Height (mAU)	Area (mAU × min)
38.59	Antcin H	0.06	0.01
43.01	Dehydrosulphurenic acid,	2.41	0.95
50.50	Eburicoic acid	1.44	0.73
59.65	Methyl antcinate B	2.01	0.65
74.07	Dehydroeburicoic acid	1.22	0.53

Table 1.
HPLC analyzed results of A. cinnamomea *extract in comparison to the purified triterpene standard.*

Cleanser and then sprayed with 3 M Cavilon™ No Sting Barrier Film solution with or without *A. cinnamomea* triterpenes.

Five experiment groups, including: 1. control mice, sprayed with 3 M Cavilon™ No Sting Barrier Film, 2. diabetic mice, sprayed with 3 M Cavilon™ No Sting Barrier Film, 3. diabetes mice, sprayed with 5 mg/kg triterpenes with 3 M Cavilon™ No Sting Barrier Film, 4. diabetic mice sprayed with 10 mg/kg triterpenes with 3MCavilon™ No Sting Barrier Film, and 5. diabetic mice sprayed with 20 mg/kg triterpenes with 3MCavilon™ No Sting Barrier Film. The wound recovery assay was observed by area change of wound healing appearance. The surgical wound area observation of the five groups was as shown in **Figure 12** (on the left).

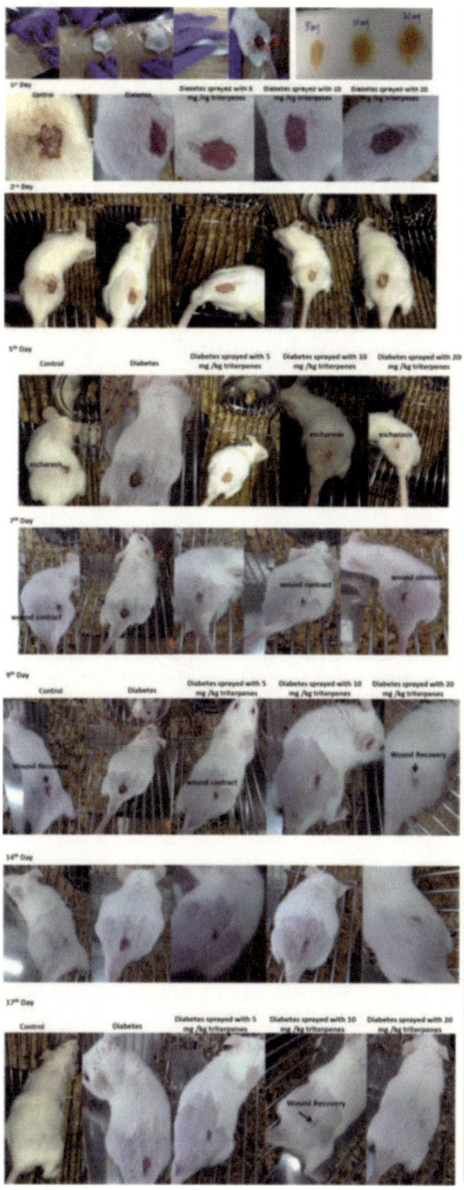

Groups / Time	Control (3 mouse)	Diabetes Mouse (3 mouse)	Diabetes Mouse Sprayed with 5 mg/kg triterpenes (3 mouse)	Diabetes Mouse Sprayed with 10 mg/kg triterpenes (3 mouse)	Diabetes Mouse Sprayed with 20 mg/kg triterpenes (3 mouse)
1st Day	Wound	Wound	Wound	Wound	Wound
2nd Day	Wound (increased wound exudate)	Wound (increased wound exudate)	Wound (increased wound exudate)	Wound (increased wound exudate)	Wound (increased wound exudate)
3rd Day	Wound (increased wound exudate)	Wound (increased wound exudate)	Wound (increased wound exudate)	Wound (increased wound exudate)	Wound (increased wound exudate)
4th Day	Wound (increased wound exudate)	Wound (increased wound exudate)	Wound (increased wound exudate)	Wound (increased wound exudate)	Wound (increased wound exudate)
5th Day	Escharosis	Wound (increased wound exudate)	Escharosis	Escharosis	Escharosis
6th Day	Escharosis	Wound	Escharosis	Escharosis	Escharosis
7th Day	Wound contract	Wound	Escharosis	wound contract	wound contract
8th Day	Wound contract	Wound	Escharosis	Wound contract	Wound contract
9th Day	Wound Recovery (Hair not totally Overlap)	Wound	Wound contract	Wound contract	Wound Recovery (Hair not totally Overlap)
10th Day	Wound Recovery (Hair not totally Overlap)	Wound	Wound contract	Wound contract	Wound Recovery (Hair not totally Overlap)
11th Day	Hair Overlap	Wound	Wound contract	Wound contract	Hair Overlap
12th Day	Hair Overlap	Wound	Wound contract	Wound contract	Hair Overlap
13th Day	Hair Overlap	Wound	Wound contract	Wound contract	Hair Overlap
14th Day	Hair Overlap	Wound	Wound contract	Wound contract	Hair Overlap
15th Day	Hair Overlap	Wound	Wound contract	Wound contract	Hair Overlap
16th Day	Hair Overlap	Wound	Wound contract	Wound contract	Hair Overlap
17th Day	Complete Recovery (Hair totally Overlap)	Wound	Wound contract	Wound Recovery (Hair not totally Overlap)	Hair Overlap

Figure 12.
Long-term observation of the wound healing process. (Left) The performance of wound healing appearance on mice; (Right) recovery effectiveness compared to the diabetes group.

The presented result as shown in the control group (without diabetes), respectively, comparing with the diabetes mice, sprayed with 5, 10, and 20 mg/kg triterpenes is significantly different in the Days 1–17 after the surgery. In the observation of Day 1 to the Day 5, the presented data has shown that the recovery of the wounded area is markedly in the control and sprayed with 20 mg/kg triterpenes group but not in the diabetes and other treatment groups. In the control group, the recovery process is significantly observed in the Day 5 followed the surgery but the diabetes group has not shown the wound recovery situation in the Day 5. In the Day 7 observation, the wound was initiated to be contacted in the control and 20 mg/kg triterpenes group, other treatment groups were not significant presented with recovery especially the diabetes group. The long-term observation of the wound healing process can be found that the control group completely healing in the Day 17. The 20 mg/kg triterpenes group was not completely wound healing (criteria was presented as hair totally overlapped on the wound) however, the wound exactly has been gradually recovery compared to the diabetes group **Figure 12** (right).

In this study, serum biological analysis was also carried out in the five groups. After administration of different concentrations of *A. cinnamomea* triterpenes orally, concentrations of serum thrombopoietin (TPO) and CCL1 were measured by ELISA. The result showed that diabetes caused an increase in circulating thrombopoietin (TPO), but it was found that daily oral administration with various concentrations of triterpenes was exactly able to reduce the concentration of serum TPO. TPO concentration reduced especially in the oral administration with 10 mg/bw-kg, 20 mg/bw-kg groups and positive control compared to the diabetes group from the 3rd week to the end of investigation ($p < 0.01$) (**Figure 13**). Although, the effect of triterpenes on the reducing CCL1 expression

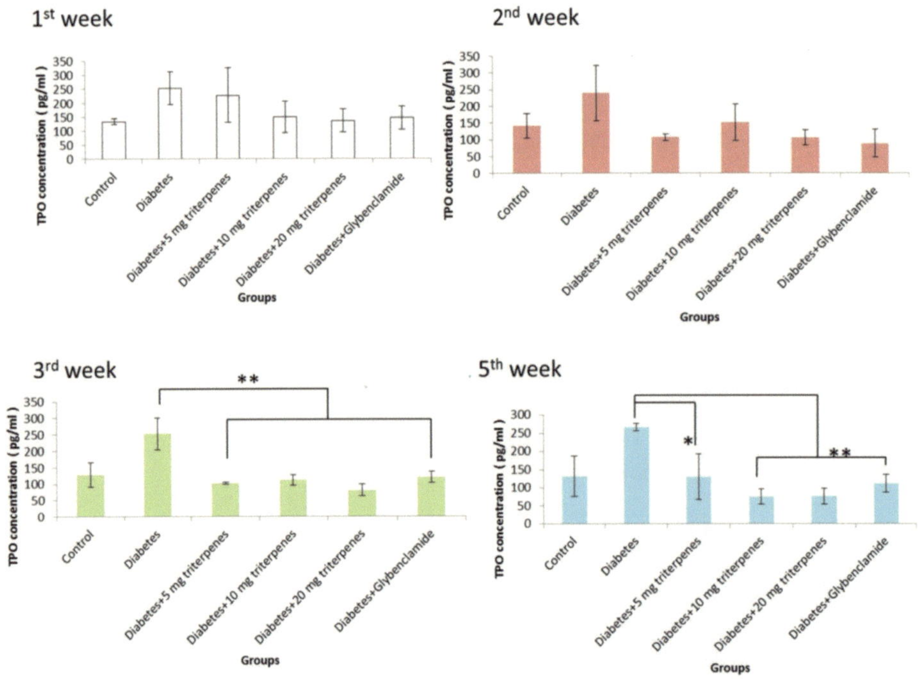

Figure 13.
Serum circulating thrombopoietin (TPO) after administration of different concentrations of A. cinnamomea *triterpenes orally in diabetic mice.*

was not significant in early observations, on continuous oral administration with various concentrations of triterpenes (10 mg/bw-kg, 20 mg/bw-kg and positive control), this effect was shown to reduce the serum CCL1 concentration in the 5th week ($p < 0.01$) (**Figure 14**).

As the result, the diabetic mice with skin wound examination, the detection of inflammatory factors such as CCL1 and TPO expression were found to induce than control mice, the hyperglycemia does cause an inflammatory response. Moreover, to the best of our knowledge, hyperglycemia impairs the tissue healing associated with an increased and prolonged inflammatory response. An investigation of the anti-inflammatory response in wound healing as affected by the triterpenes verified the promotion of wound recovery.

As the microenvironment of inflammation related to cellular transdifferentiation, migration, proliferation, survival, and extracellular matrix formation. And many factors are clearly involved in maintaining the balance between appropriate fibroblast activation and the fibrosis resulting from their continued activation for wound healing. We suggest the mechanism that the extracted triterpenes may bind to the glucocorticoid responsive elements (GREs) of target genes to regulate gene expression by mechanisms such as suppressing the expression of proinflammatory proteins and enhancing the expression of anti-inflammatory proteins. Furthermore, oleanolic acid is a triterpene that can increase insulin secretion by activating muscarinic M3 receptors in pancreatic β-cells through the Ach released from cholinergic nerve terminals. According to these findings, we suggest that the extracted triterpenes from *A. cinnamomea* may directly permeate the cell to bind with the GRE or indirectly combine with the M3 receptor, resulting in an anti-inflammatory effect and thereby promoting wound healing in the diabetic mice (**Figure 15**).

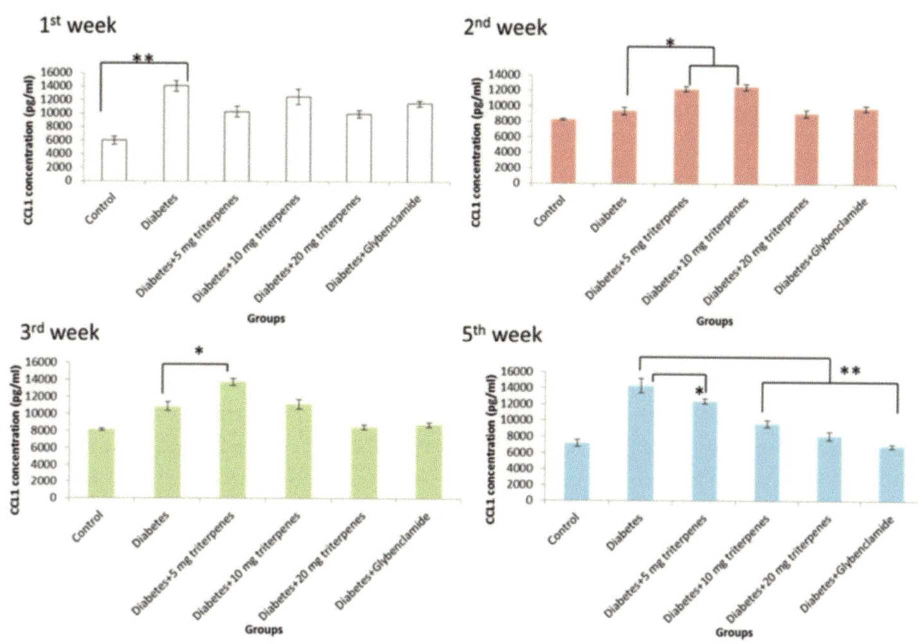

Figure 14.
Serum CCL1 after administration of different concentration A. cinnamomea *triterpenes orally in diabetic mice.*

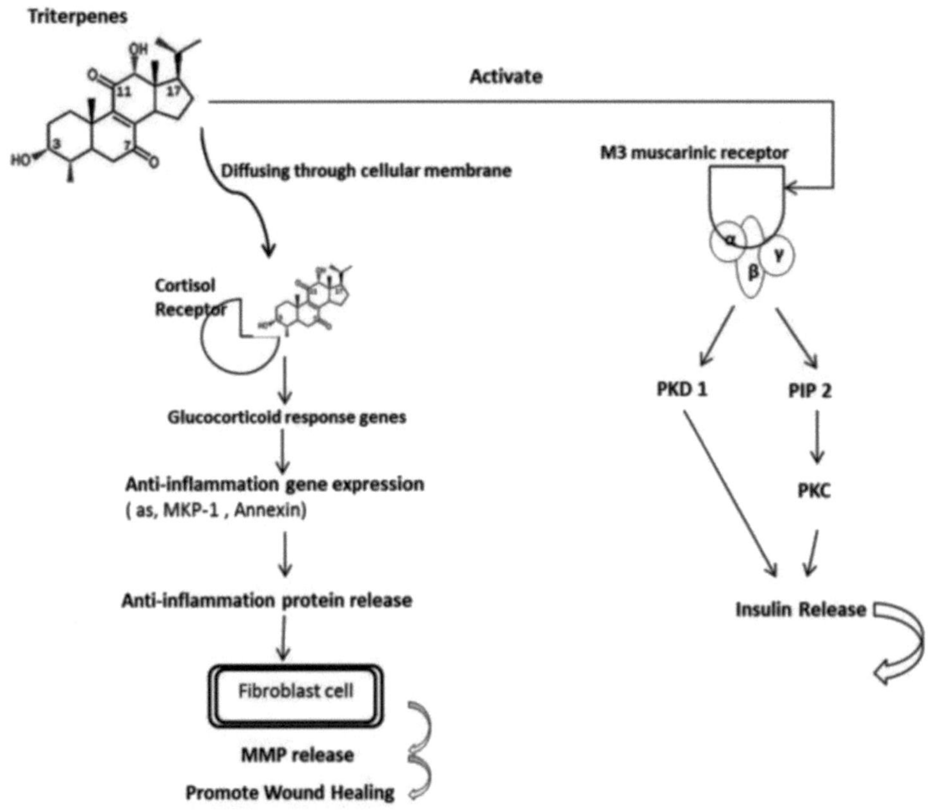

Figure 15.
The proposed mechanism of triterpenes is involved in the diabetic mice with anti-inflammation. Figure description: The mechanism of triterpenes was speculated as binding to the glucocorticoid responsive elements (GREs) of target genes to regulate gene expression such as by suppressing the expression of proinflammatory proteins and enhancing the expression of anti-inflammatory proteins. Furthermore, oleanolic acid is a triterpene that can increase insulin secretion by activating muscarinic M3 receptors in pancreatic β-cells through the Ach released from cholinergic nerve terminals. According to these findings, we suggest that the extracted triterpenes could directly permeate the cell to bind with the GRE or indirectly combine with the M3 receptor, resulting in an anti-inflammatory effect and thereby inducing wound healing in the diabetic mice.

4. A case study of the wound dressing containing mushroom β-glucan (MBG) in a type II diabetes mellitus (T2DM) patient with peripheral neuropathy

Frequent and uncontrolled hyperglycemic state from type II diabetes mellitus (T2DM) can result in peripheral neuropathy in later stages of the disease. Patients who suffer from peripheral neuropathy will often suffer from a diabetic foot that results directly from peripheral arterial disease (PAD) and/or sensory neuropathy. It is a chronic complication of T2DM. If control measures such as infections and blood glucose controls are not properly implemented, a diabetic foot can often lead to ulcers or gangrene, which eventually result in amputations.

In 2018, a patient who suffered from T2DM volunteered to be included in this case study. During the study, as shown in **Figure 16a** and **b,** the patient suffered from advanced stage of PAD, which resulted in ulcers and gangrenes on the foot's lateral and anterior sides. While the patient followed the primary physician's instructions for lifestyle alteration, routine blood glucose management as well as performing a graft surgery for the affected area, under the physician's discretion,

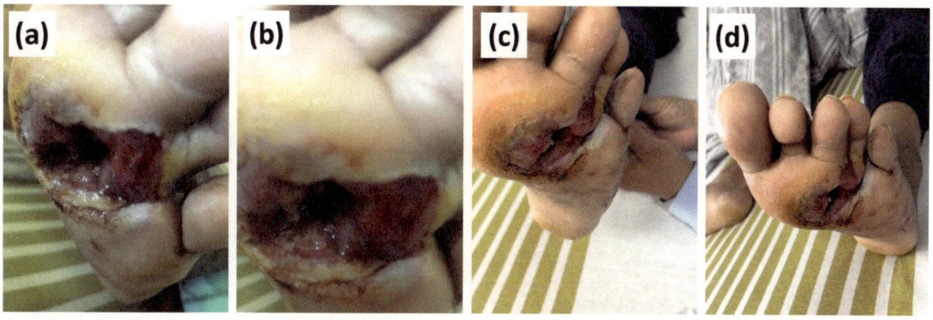

Figure 16.
The severe ulcers on diabetic patient's feet and treated with β-glucan (MBG) and triterpenes. (a, b) Gangrene resulted from peripheral arterial disease and infections. (c, d) After the test article containing G. lucidum *(Reishi) β-glucan (MBG) and triterpenes purified from A. cinnamomea applied on affected area for 2 weeks.*

a topical test article containing β-glucan isolated from *Ganoderma lucidum* (MBG) and triterpenes purified from *A. cinnamomea* was applied to the affected site three times a day (TID) as a palliative treatment to stimulate wound healing. The healing progress was recorded weekly and photographs were taken. As results show, 2 weeks after the test treatment was applied, the wounds showed a significant improvement (**Figure 16c** and **d**). From week 3 to week 10, the wounds showed even more significant improvements and the affected regions were significantly reduced (**Figure 17**). The preliminary results have demonstrated the efficacy of a powerful combination of the beta glucan and triterpenes to promote topical wound healing, that can inspire further scientific researches and applications of such in the future.

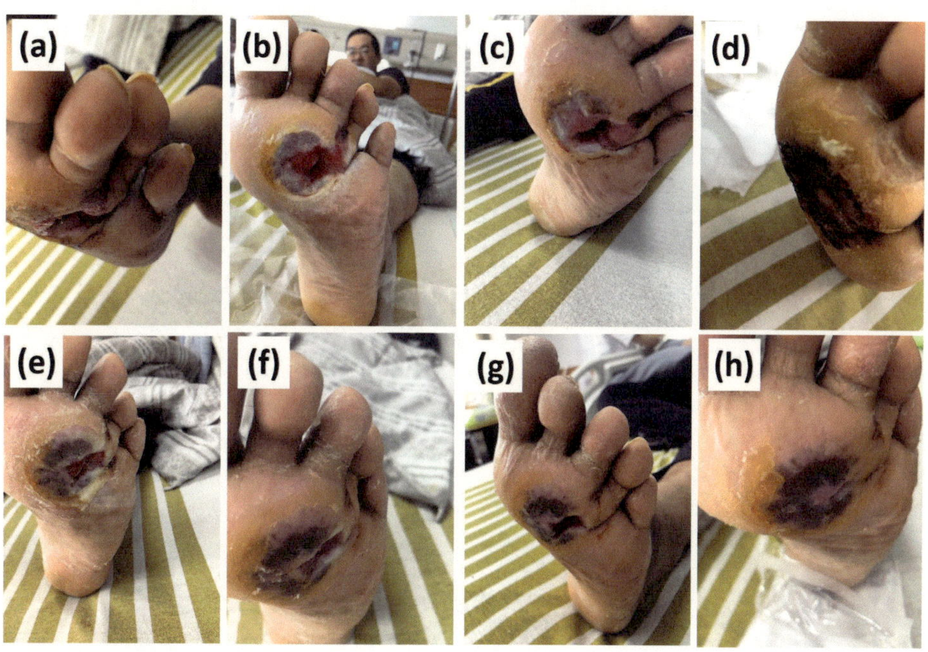

Figure 17.
A progress for diabetic patient's feet wound healing. (a–h) The healing progress of gangrenes on a T2DM patient's feet, treated by test article containing G. lucidum *(Reishi) β-glucan (MBG) and triterpenes purified from* A. cinnamomea.

Acknowledgements

The authors thank the technical services provided by the ATRI Animal Technology Laboratories to carry out wound repairing efficacy experiments on large mammals (ordinary or diabetic pigs) and the Council of Agriculture, Taiwan for funding support.

Conflict of interest

The authors declare no conflict of interest.

Author details

Shiu-Nan Chen[1], Yu-Sheng Wu[2], Sherwin Chen[1], Ya-Chin Chang[1] and Chung-Lun Lu[3]*

1 College of Life Science, National Taiwan University, Taipei, Taiwan ROC

2 Department of Aquaculture, National Pingtung University of Science and Technology, Neipu, Pingtung, Taiwan ROC

3 Aquatic Technology Laboratories, Agricultural Technology Research Institute, Hsinchu, Taiwan ROC

*Address all correspondence to: hydrocoles@msn.com

References

[1] Diabetes Mellitus. Diagnosis and classification of diabetes mellitus. Diabetes Care. 2005;**28**:37

[2] Dinh T, Elder S, Veves A. Delayed wound healing in diabetes: Considering future treatments. Diabetes Management. 2011;**1**:509-519

[3] Kuller LH. Nutrition, lipids, and cardiovascular disease. Nutrition Reviews. 2006;**64**:15-26

[4] McCowen KC, Malhotra A, Bistrian BR. Stress-induced hyperglycemia. Critical Care Clinics. 2001;**17**:107-124

[5] Nosenko MA, Ambaryan SG, Drutskaya MS. Proinflammatory cytokines and skin wound healing in mice. Molekuliarnaia Biologiia. 2019;**53**:741-754

[6] Nosenko MA, Atretkhany KN, Mokhonov VV, Vasilenko EA, Kruglov AA, Tillib SV, et al. Modulation of bioavailability of proinflammatory cytokines produced by myeloid cells. Seminars in Arthritis and Rheumatism. 2019;**49**:39-42

[7] Greenhalgh DG. Tissue repair in models of diabetes mellitus. A review. Methods in Molecular Medicine. 2003;**78**:181-189

[8] Cheng JJ, Huang NK, Chang TT, Wang DL, Lu MK. Study for anti-angiogenic activities of polysaccharides isolated from *Antrodia cinnamomea* in endothelial cells. Life Sciences. 2005;**76**:3029-3042

[9] Sen G, Khan AQ, Chen Q, Snapper CM. In vivo humoral immune responses to isolated pneumococcal polysaccharides are dependent on the presence of associated TLR ligands. Journal of Immunology. 2005;**175**:3084-3091

[10] Murphy EA, Davis JM, Carmichael MD. Immune modulating effects of beta-glucan. Current Opinion in Clinical Nutrition and Metabolic Care. 2010;**13**:656-661

[11] Lieu CW, Lee SS, Wang SY. The effect of Ganoderma lucidum on induction of differentiation in leukemic U937 cells. Anticancer Research. 1992;**12**:1211-1215

[12] Woo YI, Park BJ, Kim HL, Lee MH, Kim J, Yang YI, et al. The biological activities of (1,3)-(1,6)-beta-d-glucan and porous electrospun PLGA membranes containing beta-glucan in human dermal fibroblasts and adipose tissue-derived stem cells. Biomedical Materials. 2010;**5**. DOI: 10.1088/1748-6041/5/4/044109

[13] Hsiao CM, Wu YS, Nan FH, Huang SL, Chen L, Chen SN. Immunomodulator 'mushroom beta glucan' induces Wnt/beta catenin signalling and improves wound recovery in tilapia and rat skin: A histopathological study. International Wound Journal. 2016;**13**:1116-1128

[14] Smiderle FR, Baggio CH, Borato DG, Santana-Filho AP, Sassaki GL, Iacomini M, et al. Anti-inflammatory properties of the medicinal mushroom *Cordyceps militaris* might be related to its linear (1⟶3)-beta-D-glucan. PLoS One. 2014;**9**. DOI: 10.1371/journal.pone.0110266

[15] Suzuki Hashimoto IK, Ohno N, Tanaka H, Yadomae T. Immunomodulation by orally administered beta-glucan in mice. International Journal of Immunopharmacology. 1989;**11**:761-769

[16] Minutti CM, Knipper JA, Allen JE, Zaiss DM. Tissue-specific contribution of macrophages to wound healing. Seminars in Cell & Developmental Biology. 2017;**61**:3-11

[17] Portera CA, Love EJ, Memore L, Zhang L, Muller A, Browder W, et al. Effect of macrophage stimulation on collagen biosynthesis in the healing wound. The American Surgeon. 1997;**63**:125-131

[18] Kougias P, Wei D, Rice PJ, Ensley HE, Kalbfleisch J, Williams DL, et al. Normal human fibroblasts express pattern recognition receptors for fungal (1⟶3)-beta-D-glucans. Infection and Immunity. 2001;**69**:3933-3938

[19] Lowe EP, Wei D, Rice PJ, Li Kalbfleisch CJ, Browder IW, Williams DL. Human vascular endothelial cells express pattern recognition receptors for fungal glucans which stimulates nuclear factor kappaB activation and interleukin 8 production. Winner of the Best Paper Award from the Gold Medal Forum. The American Surgeon. 2002;**68**:508-517

[20] Lee SB, Jeon HW, Lee YW, Lee YM, Song KW, Park MH, et al. Bio-artificial skin composed of gelatin and (1⟶3), (1⟶6)-beta-glucan. Biomaterials. 2003;**24**:2503-2511

[21] Czop JK, Valiante NM, Janusz MJ. Phagocytosis of particulate activators of the human alternative complement pathway through monocyte beta-glucan receptors. Progress in Clinical and Biological Research. 1987;**297**:287-296

[22] Delatte SJ, Evans J, Hebra A, Adamson W, Othersen HB, Tagge EP. Effectiveness of beta-glucan collagen for treatment of partial-thickness burns in children. Journal of Pediatric Surgery. 2011;**36**:113-118

[23] Patel S, Goyal A. Recent developments in mushrooms as anti-cancer therapeutics: A review. 3 Biotech. 2012;**2**:1-15

[24] Chen TI, Chen CC, Lin TW, Tsai YT, Nam MK. A 90-day subchronic toxicological assessment of Antrodia cinnamomea in Sprague-Dawley rats. Food and Chemical Toxicology. 2011;**49**:429-433

[25] Geethangili M, Tzeng YM. Review of pharmacological effects of *Antrodia camphorata* and its bioactive compounds, Evidence-based complementary and alternative medicine. eCAM. 2011. DOI: 10.1093/ecam/nep108

[26] Hsu JH, Wu YC, Liu IM, Cheng JT. Release of acetylcholine to raise insulin secretion in Wistar rats by oleanolic acid, one of the active principles contained in *Cornus officinalis*. Neuroscience Letters. 2006;**404**:112-116

[27] Agra LC, Ferro JN, Barbosa FT, Barreto E. Triterpenes with healing activity: A systematic review. The Journal of Dermatological Treatment. 2015;**26**:465-470

[28] Byun-McKay A, Godard KA, Toudefallah M, Martin DM, Alfaro R, King J, et al. Wound-induced terpene synthase gene expression in Sitka spruce that exhibit resistance or susceptibility to attack by the white pine weevil. Plant Physiology. 2006;**140**:1009-1021

[29] Minns LA, Buzoni-Gatel D, Ely KH, Rachinel N, Luangsay S, Kasper LH. A novel triterpenoid induces transforming growth factor beta production by intraepithelial lymphocytes to prevent ileitis. Gastroenterology. 2004;**127**:119-126

[30] Wu YS, Chen SN. Extracted triterpenes from *Antrodia cinnamomea* reduce the inflammation to promote the wound healing via the STZ inducing Hyperglycemia-diabetes mice model. Frontiers in Pharmacology. 2016;7. DOI: 10.3389/fphar.2016.00154

[31] Peter G, Kilk R, Mokry M, Vidinsky B, Vasilenko T, Mozes S, et al. Simple method of open skin wound healing model in corticosteroid-treated and diabetic rats: Standardization of semi-quantitative and quantitative histological assessments. Veterinarni Medicina. 2008;**53**:652-659

Chapter 7

Assessment of Diabetic Foot through the Developmental Stages of Lower Limb Abnormalities Using Ultrasound

Suresh K.S. and Sukesh Kumar A.

Abstract

A diabetic foot is one of the most serious complications of diabetes mellitus. This causes large number of lower leg amputations worldwide. Usually this disease is getting diagnosed in a very later stage. Ankle-arm index, diastolic blood pressure, fasting plasma glucose, hemoglobin A1C, high blood pressure, medial arterial calcification, nerve conduction velocity, peripheral vascular disease, systolic blood pressure, transcutaneous oxygen tension, etc. are some of the major indicators of a diabetic foot. Among these peripheral arterial abnormalities and neuropathy are the most dominant visible factors. Detection and monitoring of diabetic foot help to demonstrate the feet at risk of ulceration positively. This study reveals the various assessment methodologies of lower limb abnormalities leading to diabetic foot using ultrasound. Ultrasound is being used in various cases related to diabetic foot, from the identification of systolic pressure for the ankle brachial pressure index to the velocity analysis of hemodynamic studies. The study analyses the lower limb abnormalities and extracts the features of diabetic foot from the velocity spectrum of ultrasound Doppler scan.

Keywords: diabetic foot, diabetic neuropathy, peripheral arterial disease, diabetes mellitus, early detection, Doppler ultrasound

1. Introduction

Diabetes is a growing global epidemic of the current century. This occurs either when the pancreas does not produce enough insulin or when the body cannot effectively use the produced insulin. According to the International Diabetes Federation, it is estimated that presently 387 million people are being affected by diabetes, and this may increase to 592 million in the coming 20 years [1]. In addition to this, 316 million people are at high risk with impaired glucose tolerance, and a projection shows that in 2035, the count of high-risk people will attain more than 1 billion. According to the recent estimation of the World Health Organization (WHO), diabetes is being suffered by 9% among adults aged 18+ years. Approximately 1.5 million deaths were directly caused by diabetes in 2012, and 80% of this occurred in low- and middle-income countries. Diabetes is estimated to be the seventh leading cause of death in 2030 by the WHO [2]. The statistics of the International Diabetes

Federation reveals that in India there are nearly 65 million diabetes cases [3]. The associated complications of diabetes have also been increased in proportionate to the high rate of diabetes-affected persons.

Among the variety of complications related to diabetes, a diabetic foot stands one of the most threatening one. If the foot exhibits any pathology because of diabetes mellitus or any complications due to the long-term suffering of diabetes. The study reveals various types lower limb abnormalities and analyses the features of diabetic foot from the velocity spectrum of ultrasound Doppler scan.

2. Diabetic foot disease

In diabetic cases, foot problem may develop as a part of damaging nerve and blood vessels. This may cause the infection and ulceration of the leg and finally come to the level of amputation. This is one of the dangerous conditions. Foot diseases are the most probable causes of hospital admissions in the case of diabetes. Considering the total patients suffering from diabetes mellitus, diabetic foot disease probably occurs 15–25% of them. Among the diabetic foot patients, 85% of the cases precede to partial lower leg amputation. Individuals with diabetes are 25 times bound to lose a leg than individuals without the condition.

More than 70% of leg amputations throughout the world are due to diabetes [4]. Every year, around 1 million diabetic people lose a leg because of their diseased condition. The diabetic foot also causes major economic consequences for the patients, their families and the entire society. The International Working Group on the Diabetic Foot estimated that a lower limb is lost to diabetes somewhere in the world in every 20 seconds [5].

Ankle-arm index, diastolic blood pressure, plasma glucose, hemoglobin A1C, high blood pressure, medial arterial calcification, peripheral vascular disease, systolic blood pressure and transcutaneous oxygen tension are the major identified indicators of diabetic foot. Comparing the overall visible symptoms of diabetic foot, peripheral arterial disease and diabetic neuropathy seem to be the most important threatening factors [6, 7].

3. Lower limb abnormalities leading to diabetic foot

Peripheral arterial disease (PAD) is of great clinical significance in diabetic patients. Some of them have high risk of subsequent myocardial infarction or stroke, irrespective of the presence or absence of symptoms of PAD. Lack of proper treatment can lead to functional disability and limb loss. So, regular screening of PAD is very important as a part of proper management to minimize the impact of comorbidities on the diseased person.

The human nervous system is also very much affected with diabetes. The peripheral nerves, the nerves that go to the arms, hands, legs and feet, may get damaged with persistent high glucose level. Usually, the diabetic peripheral neuropathy arises in different places of the human body but very prominently affects the sensations of the toes and feet [8]. This abnormal sensation may lead a feeling of being pricked with pins, throbbing and numbness with sharp pain and tingling and burning sensations.

The risk for foot ulcers and amputation is increased by diabetic peripheral neuropathy. People who are suffering from diabetic peripheral neuropathy mostly do not notice minor cuts, sores or blisters in their foot and toes. This is because of the loss of sensation in connection with the damage of the nerves in the corresponding areas. Neuropathy affects the sensory, motor and autonomic systems of the human body. The untreated wounds become easily infected and may lead to gangrene, which finally require amputation in that area. If this is diagnosed in the early stages, it is a major opportunity to ameliorate symptoms and prevent the development of the major clinical neuropathic endpoints of the lower limb [9] such as chronic painful foot, the insensate foot, the Charcot foot and the neuropathic ulcer. It is important that physicians and other healthcare providers understand that diabetic neuropathy can occur with no pain or with an insensate foot or may present with pain in the form of dysesthesias and paresthesias.

4. Role of ultrasound

The ultrasound wave is one of the safest and easiest modes of medical diagnosis. This modality of medical imaging helps to identify internal body structures in a noninvasive manner. This has been achieved by computerized analysis of reflected ultrasound waves. Usually frequencies of 1–30 MHz are being used for a diagnostic purpose. The resolution of the image depends on the type of wave used, higher resolution with shorter wavelengths, and the wavelength is inversely proportional to the frequency [10]. However, the use of high frequencies is limited by their greater attenuation in the tissue and thus shorter depth of penetration. The frequencies 2–10 MHz are used for vascular studies.

Doppler ultrasound provides the basis for noninvasive and objective measurements of the spectrum and serially monitors the velocity of flow in the arteries. This Doppler ultrasound has very high potential for monitoring blood flow velocity as it is reliable and noninvasive and provides real-time result. In Doppler analysis, the ultrasound beam has the sum of the instantaneous contributions of each particle crossing that beam. A human observer can interpret it because such mixtures of signals are sorted according to the frequency and weighted with the intensity in the cochlea. The signal needs to endure a similar process of sorting and weighting for visual interpretation. For this process, the Doppler signal has to be translated into the frequency domain, and it is done in real-time computation with fast Fourier transform of successive segments of the Doppler signal. The stationarity of the blood flow may be assumed by shortening the segments.

The power spectrum generated for each segment indicates the velocity distribution of the particles within that beam during the time interval in accordance with the width of the segment. The inverse of the time interval indicates the spectral resolution. Power spectrum point relates to a frequency interval showing a velocity range, whereas the height of each point signifies the power or the quantity of particles in that particular velocity range.

5. Vascular examination

The ankle-brachial pressure index (ABPI) is one of the most common techniques being used for initial diagnosis of foot disease. This is a particular ratio of the recorded highest pressure at the ankle for that leg to the highest brachial pressure measured for both arms. The normal range of ABPI comes below 1. When ABPI < 0.92, it is an indication of arterial disease. The value of ABPI between 0.5 and 0.9 may be connected with claudication, and for these symptoms the patient should be referred for further examination. If ABPI rate is below 0.5, it is a symptom of severe arterial disease, and this may be associated with gangrene, ischemic ulceration or rest pain, and urgent referral is required for a vascular opinion. The pressure at the ankle and brachial artery is determined with the ultrasound. Pressure is measured by blood pressure apparatus, but the auscultation is determined by Doppler ultrasound [11]. The state of peripheral circulation can be easily identified with the examination of the legs. Peripheral arterial examination using ultrasound gives a lot of indications related to diabetic foot [12]. Stenosis or occlusions in the segments of the peripheral arteries can be detected in patients who have suspected arterial occlusive disease. The clinical indications such as claudication, ischemic tissue loss, rest pain and suspected arterial embolization may exist in these patients. The sites can be monitored by various percutaneous interventions, including angioplasty, thrombolysis, atherectomy, and stent placements. The examination can also be done by the evaluation of suspected vascular and perivascular abnormalities, such as aneurysms, pseudoaneurysms and arteriovenous fistulas. The presence of significant arterial abnormalities can be identified and confirmed by imaging modalities [13].

One of the indications for peripheral venous ultrasound examinations is the evaluation of possible venous thromboembolic disease or venous obstruction in symptomatic or high-risk asymptomatic individuals. Assessments of venous insufficiency, reflux and varicosities are some of the other indications. The examination is also being done by the evaluation of veins before venous access. Follow-up for patients with known venous thrombosis near the anticipated end of anticoagulation is used in the presence of residual venous thrombosis [14].

The arterial occlusive disease is identified by the evaluation of the arterial segments, such as lower extremity, common femoral artery, proximal superficial femoral artery, mid superficial femoral artery, distal superficial femoral artery, popliteal artery, etc. A focused or limited examination may be appropriate in certain clinical situations. At a minimum, an angle-corrected spectral Doppler waveform with velocity measurements should be obtained from any of the above sites. If clinically appropriate, imaging of the iliac, deep femoral, tibioperoneal and dorsalis pedis arteries can be performed [15].

Figure 1 shows the evaluation of a patient having pain in the left lower limb. The spectral color Doppler ultrasound of the venous system has been done in this case. The color Doppler images analyze the study of veins such as popliteal, left femoral and peroneal veins and anterior-posterior tibial veins.

Usually complete visualization of the veins of the leg is very difficult. Normally it is being done by imaging the upper third and distal third of the anterior, posterior tibial and peroneal veins.

Figure 2 is an ultrasound color Doppler image of the right lower limb showing early indications of diabetic arteriopathy. This is also called as diabetic vasculopathy. The corresponding characteristic features in the color Doppler ultrasound image are:

- In the arterial waveform, there is a spectral broadening from the popliteal artery downwards.
- Slight decrease in the peak systolic velocity below the popliteal artery.
- Early changes of loss of the triphasic spectral waveform are present in the peroneal artery.

The changes mentioned above are typically seen in early diabetic arteriopathy indicating mild stenosis in a diffuse fashion below the popliteal artery.

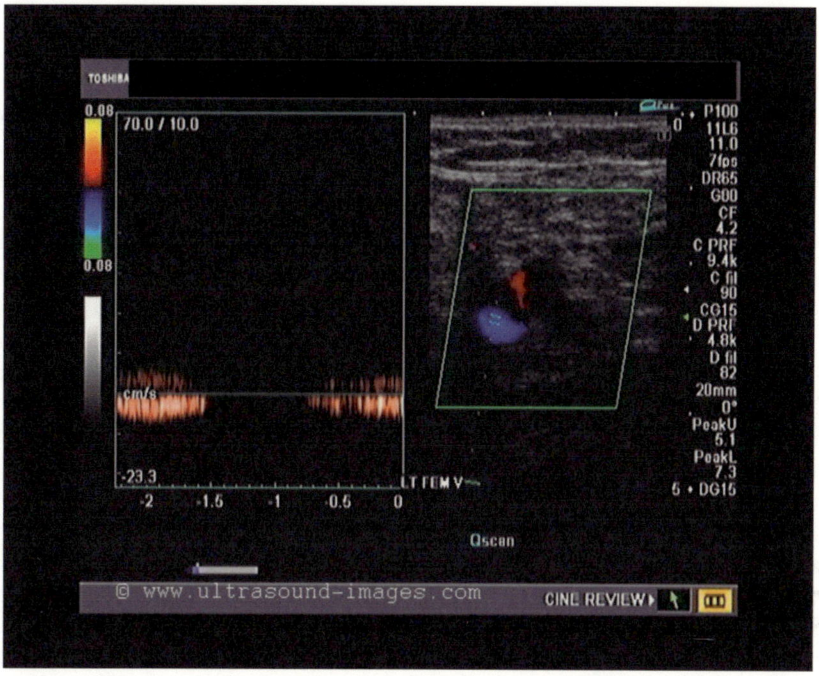

Figure 1.
Venous Doppler of the lower limb: normal case (presented with permission from Dr. Joe's ultrasound).

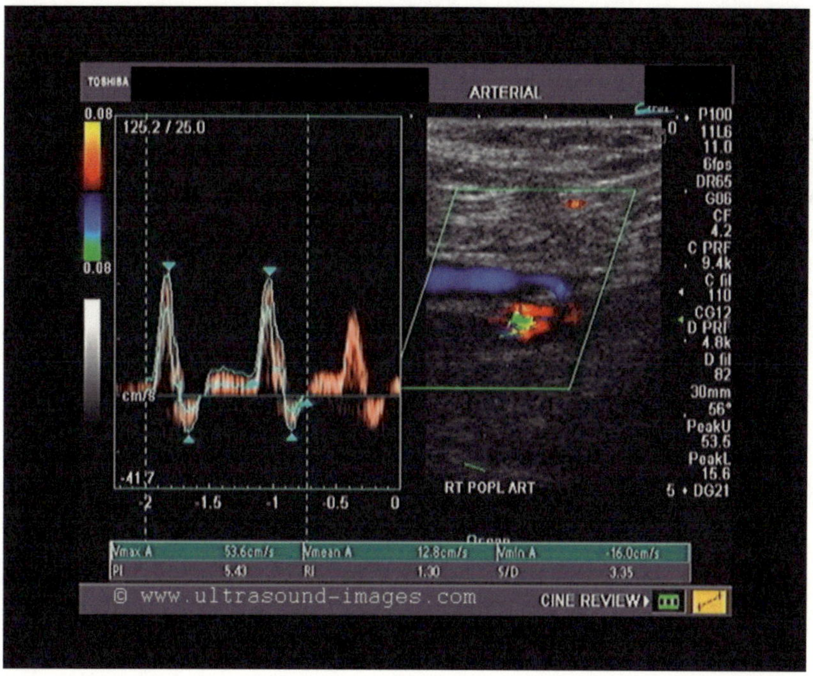

Figure 2.
Mild diabetic arteriopathy of the lower limb (presented with permission from Dr. Joe's ultrasound scan, Cochin).

In Doppler waveform analysis, normal pulsed wave is a clearly defined tracing with narrow Doppler spectrum. In normal cases, the peripheral artery waveform is triphasic. When blood flow becomes turbulent at bifurcations and luminal narrowing, it causes spectral broadening of Doppler waveform.

6. Velocity spectrum

The Doppler arterial waveform images can be analyzed to provide information about blood flow in or out of the gut and related along with the other physiological measurements.

The velocity information perceived from a single location in the blood vessel is displayed in the form of frequency shift-time plot in the case of real-time spectral Doppler analysis. The time along the horizontal axis and frequency shift or identified velocity along the vertical axis will be displayed.

The clinical information attained from the maximum Doppler shift correspond to a spatial maximum in the velocity field. Systematic analysis can be done with spectral Doppler ultrasound velocimetry, an analysis of the spectrum of frequencies by which the Doppler signal is constituted [16].

The Doppler frequency shift happens with backscattering of millions of red blood cells. The resultant shifted signal is the summation of such multiple Doppler frequency shifts.

The processing of Doppler signal is accomplished through various steps. After the initial reception, the next step is amplification. It is demodulated, and the characteristic parameters of flow are identified by further spectral processing methods. The Doppler shift frequency is proportional to the velocity of the blood flow. The power in a particular frequency band of the Doppler spectrum is proportional to the volume of blood, under ideal uniform sampling conditions.

As the blood moving with velocities create frequencies in the particular band, the power Doppler spectrum has the same shape as the velocity distribution plot for the flow in the vessel. The deviation in the shape of the Doppler power spectrum as a function of time is normally denoted in the form of sonograms.

7. Conclusion

The frequency level and patterns of lower limb arterial insufficiency in diabetic patients can be evaluated by Doppler-based techniques. The most prominent case of diabetic foot is the development of vasculopathic changes leading to peripheral vascular insufficiency. This can be detected by analyzing velocity spectrum of blood flow in the lower limb. Angle-corrected spectral Doppler waveforms should be effectively utilized for the recognition procedure. Precise evaluation has to be attained with further analysis.

Acknowledgements

We are very much thankful to Dr. Joe's Ultrasound Scan, Cochin, and Niranjan Ultrasound India (P) Ltd., Calicut, for providing clinical support for this research work.

Author details

Suresh K.S.[1*] and Sukesh Kumar A.[2]

1 Centre for Development of Imaging Technology, Thiruvananthapuram, Kerala, India

2 Rajiv Gandhi Institute of Development Studies, Thiruvananthapuram, India

*Address all correspondence to: sureshkstvm05@gmail.com

References

[1] International Diabetes Federation, Annual Report; 2014

[2] World Health Organization. Diabetes Programme. 2015. Available from: http://www.who.int/diabetes/en/

[3] International Diabetes Federation. IDF Diabetes Atlas. 6th ed; 2013. Available from: http://www.idf.org/diabetesatlas

[4] International Diabetes Federation. Diabetes and Foot Care Time to Act; 2005

[5] International Working Group on the Diabetic Foot. Guidance docsuments. 2015. Available from: http://iwgdf.org/guidelines/

[6] Reiber GE, Lemaster JW. Epidemiology and economic impact of foot ulcers and amputations in people with diabetes. In: Levin and O'Neal's the Diabetic Foot. 7th ed. USA: Mosby Elsevier PA; 2008. pp. 3-22

[7] Zimny S, Dessel F, Ehren M, Pfohl M. Helmut Schatz "early detection of microcirculatory impairment in diabetic patients with foot at risk". Diabetes Care. 2001;**24**:1810-1814

[8] Suresh KS, Sukesh Kumar A. An investigation for early stage diagnosis of diabetic foot. International Journal of Enhanced Research In Science Technology & Engineering. 2016;**5**(12):40-43

[9] Suresh KS, Sukesh Kumar A. Clinical need of a diabetic foot infection detector. In: National Conference on Advances in Computational Intelligence & Communication Technologies. 2016. pp. 125-128

[10] World Health Organization. Manual of Diagnostic Ultrasound; 2011

[11] Suresh KS, Sukesh Kumar A. An integrated model for early detection and monitoring of diabetic foot. In: Proceedings of International Conference on Modelling and Simulation, Association for the Advancement of Modelling and Simulation Techniques in Enterprises. 2017

[12] Bessonov N, Sequeira A, Simakov S, Vassilevskii Y, Volpert V. Methods of blood flow modelling. Mathematical Modelling of Natural Phenomena. 2016;**11**(1):1-25

[13] Lingegowda D, Moorthy S, Sreekumar KP, Kannan RR. Imaging in diabetic ischemic foot. International Journal of Diabetes in Developing Countries. 2010;**30**(4):179-184

[14] AIUM Practice Guide Line for the Performance of Peripheral Venous Ultrasound Examinations. American Institute of Ultrasound in Medicine; 2010

[15] AIUM Practice Guide Line for the Performance of Peripheral Arterial Ultrasound Examinations Using Color and Spectral Doppler Imaging. American Institute of Ultrasound in Medicine; 2010

[16] Gerhard-Herman M, Gardin JM, Jaff M, Mohler E, Roman M, Naqvi TZ. Guidelines for noninvasive vascular laboratory testing: A report from the American Society of Echocardiography and the Society of Vascular Medicine and Biology. Journal of the American Society of Echocardiography. 2006;**19**(8):955-972

Chapter 8

Chronic Limb-Threatening Ischemia (CLTI) in Diabetic Patients: Looking at the Big Picture beyond Wound, Ischemia and Foot Infection (WIfI) Classification System

Maria Pilar Vela-Orús and María Sonia Gaztambide-Sáenz

Abstract

During the 1990s, most diabetic ulcers were considered neuropathic, but the Eurodiale study showed that more than 50% of these were non-plantar (neuro-ischaemic and ischaemic). According to the International Guidelines, the neuro-ischaemic and ischaemic diabetic foot ulcer (DFU) outcomes are connected to factors related to the wound, leg-associated factors and patients' comorbidities. We used wound, ischaemia and foot infection (WIfI) classification system; Trans-Atlantic Inter-Society Consensus-II (TASC-II) arterial lesion score; and Kaiser Permanente pyramid (stratification of patients according to their complexity) for assessing these parameters. From February 2011 to June 2012, we collected 124 episodes of neuro-ischaemic and ischaemic active ulcer in 100 patients: 18 required major amputation, 14 of them were in WIfI stage 4 and 4 in WIfI stage 3. Ten patients (over 14 in WIfI stage 4) were classified as TASC-II D. Eight patients (over the same 14) were classified as the higher risk of Kaiser Permanente pyramid. In line with other studies, our data support that the WIfI classification correlates well regarding risk of amputation at 1 year. However, when adding TASC-II and Kaiser Permanente pyramid assessment, the outcome is even more accurate not only for limb salvage but also for patients' survival.

Keywords: critical limb ischaemia, chronic limb-threatening ischaemia, diabetic foot ulcers, diabetic foot ulcer classification systems, outcome predictors

1. Introduction

Nowadays, diabetes is considered as a leading cause of non-traumatic amputation all around the world. Despite the high morbidity and mortality associated with diseases of the foot in diabetes and although it is costly to both healthcare providers and the patient and their families [1], it is a topic that has generally failed to attract the same level of interest by healthcare professionals as other diabetes complications.

The concept of critical limb ischaemia (CLI) implies that there are objective values that inform about the perfusion below which, if we do not increase the blood supply, the limb will be lost. CLI was defined for the first time in 1982 as rest pain with ankle pressure < 40 mmHg or necrosis and ankle pressure < 60 mmHg [2]. In 2017 the European Society of Cardiology and the European Society for Vascular Surgery (ESC/ESVS) guidelines on the diagnosis and treatment of peripheral arterial disease (PAD) have replaced the term critical limb ischaemia with chronic limb-threatening ischaemia (CLTI). The authors gave three arguments for this change: first, not all patients are in a "critical" situation even if they are not revascularized. Second, due to change in the population affected, mostly diabetics with neuro-ischaemic ulcers, it was recognized that severe ischaemia was not the only underlying cause. And finally, the risk of amputation does not only depend on the extent of ischaemia but also on the presence of wound and infection [3].

According to the World Health Organization (WHO), the diabetic foot may be defined as a group of syndromes in which neuropathy, ischaemia and infection lead to tissue breakdown, resulting in morbidity, possible amputation and mortality [4].

It is admitted that ischaemic and neuro-ischaemic ulcers have similar behaviour to each other compared to the neuropathic ones referred to major amputation and survival [5].

Before the Eurodiale study, published in 2007 [6], it was widely believed that most diabetic ulcers were neuropathic, but this study found that:

- More than 50% (52%) of the foot ulcers were non-plantar (ischaemic and neuro-ischaemic).
- More than 50% (58%) of patients with an ulcer had signs of infection.
- One third of the patients (31%) had signs of both peripheral arterial disease and infection. These patients have a worse prognosis; they take longer to heal and have more amputations and more risk of dying. They have a distinct profile: they are older and have more non-plantar ulcers, greater tissue loss and more serious comorbidities.

The results from the Eurodiale study underlined that not only ulcer healing depends on the wound, the limb and the patient, but also the future of the extremity and patient survival too.

The International Guidelines [7] have published similar results: the neuro-ischaemic and ischaemic diabetic ulcer outcome is connected to:

- Factors related to the wound (the most important is the extent of tissue involvement).
- Limb-related factors (in these cases severity of PAD).
- Patients' comorbidities (see **Figure 1**).

Apelqvist in 1151 patients with diabetes and CLTI confirmed the three above-mentioned factors. Moreover, revascularization is the major driver for ulcer healing. In fact, both percutaneous transluminal angioplasty (PTA) and open vascular surgery increased the probability for primary healing with an odds ratio (OR) of 1.77 and 2.05, respectively [8].

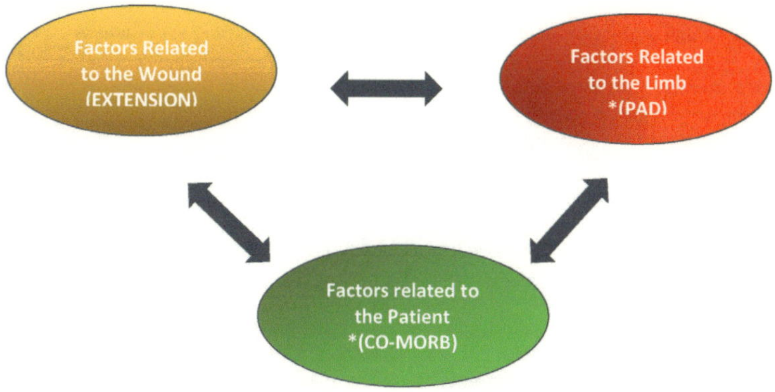

Figure 1.
*Contributors to the neuro-ischaemic and ischaemic diabetic foot ulcers (DFUs) outcomes. *PAD, peripheral arterial disease; **CO-MORB, comorbidities.*

However, data about natural history of the disease are scarce. Elgzyri in 602 patients with diabetic foot ulcer (DFU) who had been considered as CLTI and were not revascularized reported that [9]:

- 50% healed primarily with wound care or with minor amputation
- 17% healed, but after a major amputation
- 33% died with limbs intact but with unhealed wounds

1.1 Multidisciplinary team approach

Dr. Joslin, the famous American diabetologist, observed that after the introduction of insulin, "the mortality from diabetic coma had fallen dramatically (from 60 to 5%) yet deaths from diabetic gangrene of the foot and leg had risen significantly". He believed that diabetic gangrene was preventable and his remedy was a team approach involving nurses, surgeons and podiatrists for limb salvage and foot care. He was also the first to advocate for teaching patients to care for their own diabetes and the first who named diabetes as a serious public health issue that was becoming a pandemic [10].

Dr. Edmonds in 1979 in UK recognized the need for coordinated intensive care of patients with diabetic foot with input from several disciplines, including diabetology, medicine, orthopedics and vascular surgery as well as podiatrists, orthotists and nurses. This initiative resulted in an immediate 50% reduction in major amputations (1984). Specific emphasis was placed on podiatric debridement, off-loading, infection control and diabetes care [11].

The diabetic rapid response acute foot team (DRRAFT) guidelines [12], published in 2009, suggest that the vascular surgeon and diabetic podiatrist constitute the minimum in the formation of a diabetic foot team.

The authors defined seven vital skills for such a team to be able to effectively manage the lower-extremity complications of diabetes (see **Table 1**).

The Multidisciplinary Diabetic Foot Unit (MDFU) was introduced at our institution in February 2011. The team was working in three levels of care: primary prevention, acute patients' treatment and outpatient postoperative management. Day-to-day care was carried out by a podiatrist and a vascular surgeon, the basic American "toe and flow" approach [13]. An algorithm for urgent referral was introduced in our Unit regarding the ulcer, the leg and the patient (see **Figure 2**).

Haemodynamic and anatomic vascular assessment with revascularization, as necessary
Biomechanical and podiatric assessment with surgical and non-surgical intervention as necessary
Peripheral neurological examinations
Wound assessment and staging/grading of infection and ischaemia
Site-specific bedside and intraoperative incisions and debridement, taking samples for culture using an appropriate technique
Initiate and modify culture-specific and patient-appropriate antibiotic therapy
Conduct appropriate postoperative monitoring to reduce risks of re-ulceration

Table 1.
Minimum skills for constituting a diabetic foot team from DRRAFT [12].

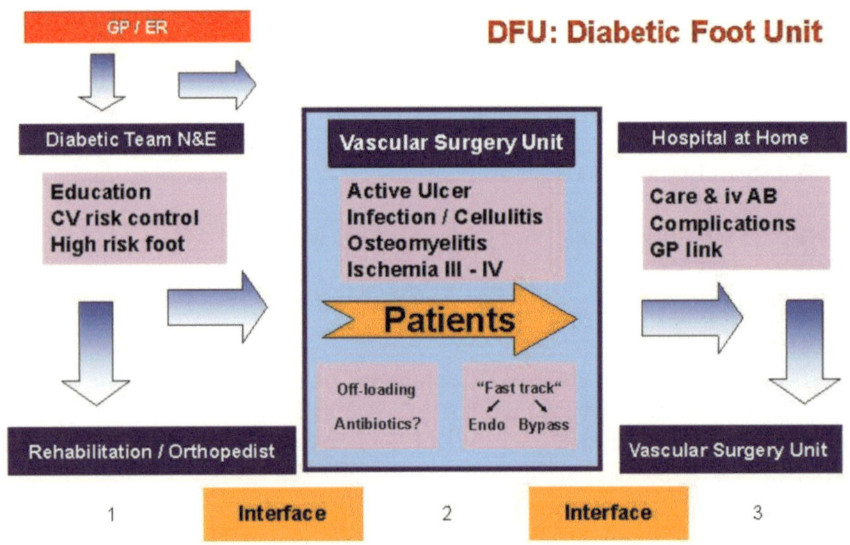

Figure 2.
Multidisciplinary diabetic foot unit organization (toe and flow inspired). GP, general practitioner; ER, emergency room; N&E, nurses and endocrinologist; CV, cardio vascular; iv AB, intravenous antibiotics.

1.2 Understanding diabetic foot ulcer classifications

Classifications that we use in daily clinical practice are compartmentalized: some refer only to infection, and others only to ischaemia or only treat descriptive aspect of ulcers [14] (see **Table 2**).

Monteiro-Soares in a meta-analysis published in 2014 identified 25 different classification systems for diabetic foot ulcers. Of those, eight used a descriptive basis, and seven utilized prognostic stratification classification systems, but few studies evaluated their reliability or external validity [15].

The International Working Group on Diabetic Foot (IWGDF) has published in 2019 his updated guidelines on the prevention and management of diabetic foot disease with a new and special chapter focus on the classification of active diabetic foot ulcers. The authors identified eight key factors judged to contribute to the scoring of classifications: some are patient-related (e.g., end-stage renal failure

Classification system	Main points	Pros/cons
Meggitt-Wagner	Assesses ulcer depth plus the presence of gangrene and loss of perfusion using six grades (0–5)	Well established Conversely, infection and ischaemia are not fully addressed
Texas University	Assesses ulcer depth, infection and ischaemia using a matrix of four grades combined with four stages	Well established Describes infection and ischaemia better than Meggitt-Wagner but informs only about yes or no (is not categorized). May help in predicting the outcome of DFUs
PEDIS Perfusion, extent (size), depth (tissue loss), infection and sensation (neuropathy)	Developed by IWGDF Uses four grades (1–4)	User-friendly (clear definitions, few categories) for practitioners with a lower level of experience with diabetic foot management
SINBAD Site, ischaemia, neuropathy, bacterial infection, area and depth	It grades area, depth, infection arteriopathy and neuropathy and site. Uses a scoring system to help predict outcomes and enable comparisons between different settings and countries	Simplified version of the S (AD) SAD classification system. Includes ulcer site as data suggests this might be an important determinant of outcome

Table 2.
Pros and cons of some common wound classification systems for DFUs [14].

Clinical scenario	Classification recommended
Communication among health professionals	*SINBAD
Predicting the outcome of an individual ulcer	None
Assessment of infection	**IDSA/IWGDF#
Assessment of perfusion and the likely benefit of revascularization	WIfI##
Audit of outcome in local, regional or national populations	SINBAD

**SINBAD, site, ischaemia, neuropathy, bacterial infection, area and depth.*
***IDSA, Infectious Diseases Society of America.*
#IWGDF, International Working Group on Diabetic Foot.
##WIfI, Wound, Ischaemia and foot Infection.

Table 3.
IWGDF classification system recommendations [16].

(ESRF)); others, limb-related (e.g., PAD and loss of protective sensation) and lastly ulcer-related (area, depth, site, single or multiple and infection). They identified five clinical key situations too and recommended one specific classification for each one: communication among health professionals; predicting the outcome of an individual ulcer; aid to clinical decision-making for an individual case; assessment of a wound, with or without infection, and peripheral artery disease; and audit of outcome in local, regional or national populations [16–18] (see **Tables 3–5**).

In order for a stratification system of a disease to be relevant, it is expected that it will give us a risk scale with respect to natural history and that the classification is detailed enough to compare different treatments. Thus, the scale could be descriptive and predictive at the same time. In January 2014 the Society for Vascular Surgery (SVS) published the new classification system for CLTI based on wound extent, degree of ischaemia and foot infection (WIfI), with scales from 0 to 3, for each one of these parameters [19].

Category	Definition	Score
Site	Forefoot	0
	Midfoot and hindfoot	1
Ischemia	Pedal blood flow intact (at least one palpable pulse)	0
	Clinical evidence of reduced pedal flow	1
Neuropathy	Protective sensation intact	0
	Protective sensation lost	1
Bacterial infection	None	0
	Present	1
Area	Ulcer <1 cm^2	0
	Ulcer >1 cm^2	1
Depth	Ulcer confined to the skin and subcutaneous tissue	0
	Ulcer reaching the muscle, tendon or deeper	1
Total possible score		6

Table 4.
SINBAD classification system [17].

Clinical manifestations	Infection severity	PEDIS grade
Wound lacking purulence or any manifestations of inflammation	Uninfected	1
Presence of >2 manifestations of inflammation (purulence, erythema, tenderness, warmth or induration), but any cellulitis/erythema extends <2 cm around the ulcer, and the infection is limited to the skin or superficial subcutaneous tissues; no other local complications or systemic illness	Mild	2
Infection (as above) in a patient who is systemically well and metabolically stable but which has >1 of the following characteristics: cellulitis extending >2 cm, lymphangitic streaking, spread beneath the superficial fascia, deep tissue abscess, gangrene and involvement of muscle, tendon, joint or bone	Moderate	3
Infection in a patient with systemic toxicity or metabolic instability (e.g. fever, chills, tachycardia, hypotension, confusion, vomiting, leukocytosis, acidosis, severe hyperglycemia or azotemia)	Severe	4

Table 5.
IDSA/IWGDF system [18].

WIfI classification represents a summary of multiple previously published classifications focused on diabetic foot ulcers and pure ischaemia or infection models and is the first one which reports on the risk of amputation and benefit of revascularization at 1 year.

With respect to the wound, WIfI integrates the Texas University classification that is validated and adds the gangrene component. The authors include pain at rest and gangrene of ischaemic cause. Depth takes preference over extension, and there is a measure of what is going to lose (see **Table 6**).

WIfI ischaemia is stratified not only according to ankle-brachial index (ABI) figures but also ankle pressure and digital pressure. They are categorized up to moderate degrees of ischaemia. Alternatives to the ABI are included, and digital pressure is considered mandatory in diabetic patients (see **Table 7**).

WIfI collects the characteristics of the Infectious Diseases Society of America (IDSA) (validated) and the IWGDF (see **Table 8**).

Based on the results obtained in each parameter, a Delphi survey among 12 experts was conducted. A table for estimating the risk of major amputation over the first year and the theoretical benefit of revascularization was elaborated.

Wound grade	Diabetic foot ulcer (DFU)	Gangrene
0	No ulcer Clinical description: minor tissue loss (1 or 2 digits)	No gangrene Salvageable with simple digital amputation or skin coverage
1	Small, shallow ulcer(s) on distal leg or foot; no exposed bone, unless limited to the distal phalanx Clinical description: minor tissue loss (1 or 2 digits)	No gangrene Salvageable with simple digital amputation or skin coverage
2	Deeper ulcer with exposed bone, joint or tendon; generally, not involving the heel; shallow heel ulcer, without calcaneal involvement Clinical description: major tissue loss	Gangrenous changes limited to digits Salvageable with multiple (>3) digital amputation or standard trans-metatarsal amputation (TMA) ± skin coverage
3	Extensive, deep ulcer involving the forefoot and/or midfoot; deep full-thickness heel ulcer ± calcaneal involvement Clinical description: extensive tissue loss	Extensive gangrene involving the forefoot and/or midfoot; full-thickness heel necrosis and calcaneal involvement Salvageable only with a complex foot reconstruction or non-traditional TMA (Chopart or Lisfranc) flap coverage or complex wound management needed for large soft tissue defect

Table 6.
Wound from WIfI system [19].

Ischemia grade	Ankle-brachial index	Ankle systolic pressure (mmHg)	Toe pressure, trans-cutaneous oxygen pressure (mmHg)
0	>0.80	>100	>60
1	0.6–0.79	70–100	40–59
2	0.4–0.59	50–70	30–39
3	<0.39	<50	<30

Table 7.
Ischemia from WIfI system [19].

Foot infection grade	Clinical manifestations
0	No symptoms or signs of infection Infection present, as defined by the presence of at least 2 of the following items: local swelling or induration; erythema >0.5 to <2 cm around the ulcer; local tenderness or pain; local warmth; purulent discharge: thick, opaque to white or sanguineous secretion
1	Local infection involving only the skin and the subcutaneous tissue (without involvement of deeper tissues and without systemic signs as described below). Exclude other causes of an inflammatory response of the skin (e.g. trauma, gout, acute Charcot, neuro-osteoarthropathy, fracture, thrombosis, venous stasis)
2	Local infection (as described above) with erythema >2 cm, or involving structures deeper than the skin and subcutaneous tissues (e.g. abscess, osteomyelitis, septic arthritis, fasciitis), and no systemic inflammatory response signs (as described below)
3	Local infection (as described above) with the signs of SIRS, as manifested by two or more of the following: temperature > 38°C or < 36°C; heart rate > 90 beats/min; respiratory rate > 20 breaths/min or PaCO2 < 32 mmHg; white blood cell count >12,000 or < 4000 cu/mm or 10% immature (band) forms

Table 8.
Foot infection from WIfI system [19].

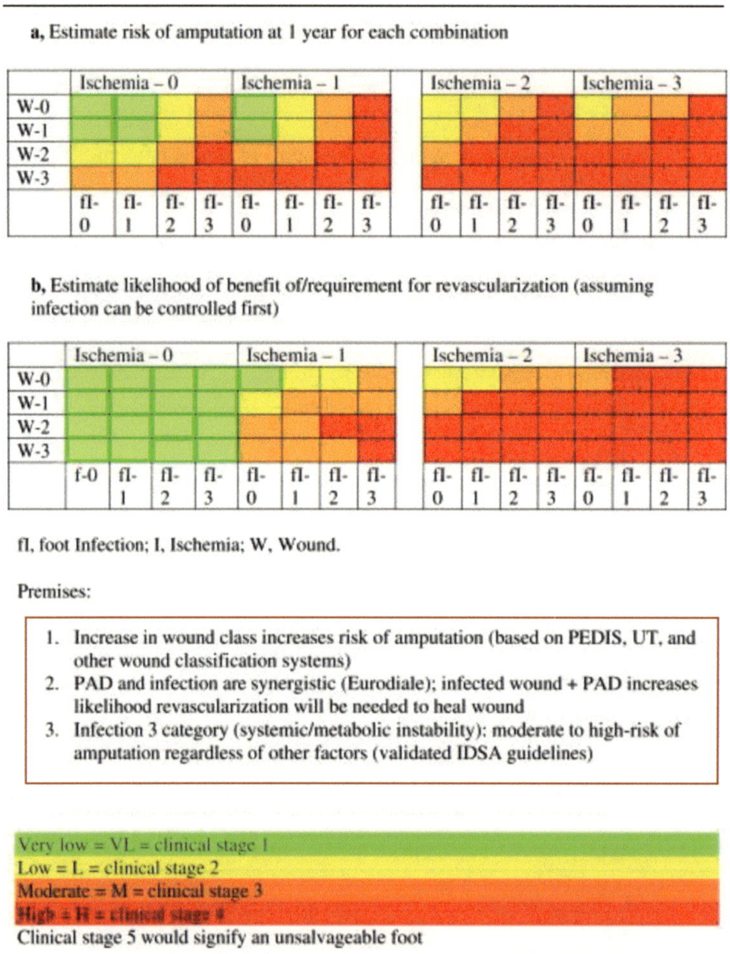

a, Estimate risk of amputation at 1 year for each combination

	Ischemia – 0				Ischemia – 1				Ischemia – 2				Ischemia – 3			
W-0																
W-1																
W-2																
W-3																
	fI-0	fI-1	fI-2	fI-3	fI-0	fI-1	fI-2	fI-3	fI-0	fI-1	fI-2	fI-3	fI-0	fI-1	fI-2	fI-3

b, Estimate likelihood of benefit of/requirement for revascularization (assuming infection can be controlled first)

	Ischemia – 0				Ischemia – 1				Ischemia – 2				Ischemia – 3			
W-0																
W-1																
W-2																
W-3																
	f-0	fI-1	fI-2	fI-3	fI-0	fI-1	fI-2	fI-3	fI-0	fI-1	fI-2	fI-3	fI-0	fI-1	fI-2	fI-3

fI, foot Infection; I, Ischemia; W, Wound.

Premises:

1. Increase in wound class increases risk of amputation (based on PEDIS, UT, and other wound classification systems)
2. PAD and infection are synergistic (Eurodiale); infected wound + PAD increases likelihood revascularization will be needed to heal wound
3. Infection 3 category (systemic/metabolic instability): moderate to high-risk of amputation regardless of other factors (validated IDSA guidelines)

Very low = VL = clinical stage 1
Low = L = clinical stage 2
Moderate = M = clinical stage 3
High = H = clinical stage 4
Clinical stage 5 would signify an unsalvageable foot

Table 9.
WIfI prediction tables. Adapted from the original [19].

When calculating the benefit of revascularization, they assume that the infection is controlled. Intraclass correlation coefficient for the amputation in the first year was 0.81/0.98 and for the benefit of revascularization 0.76/0.97 (see **Table 9**).

2. Looking at the big picture

In a recent meta-analysis published in 2019 regarding the prognostic value of the WIfI classification in patients with CLTI and where 12 studies comprising 2669 patients were evaluated, the authors conclude that “the likelihood of an amputation after 1 year in patients with CLTI increases with higher WIfI stages”. But, “the current evidence is not sufficient for the instrument to be helpful in clinical decision making for patients with CLTI and prospective studies are needed to determine its role in clinical practice” [20]. We are aware that the risk of amputation increases as the WIfI clinical stage progresses from stage 1 to stage 4. However, data regarding those with PAD and their anatomical conditions and patients’ comorbidities are lacking in WIfI classification system. By better defining and understanding CLTI spectrum, we need to include arterial lesion classification and patients’ comorbidities.

Existing systems of classification of critical ischaemia (e.g., classical Fontaine and Rutherford) do not adequately explain the extent of tissue loss or the presence and severity of infection. In recent years, most classifications have focused on anatomical details extracted from arteriography without paying attention to the physiological state of the limb, for example, the Bollinger, Graziani and Trans-Atlantic Inter-Society Consensus (TASC-I and TASC-II) classifications. Although there are criticisms, the TASC-I and TASC-II classifications are the only ones that carry recommendations for treatment [21] (see **Figure 3**). And we should also use a classification that describes the state of the arteries in the foot [22].

If we assume that in ulcer healing, factors are related not only to the wound itself but also to the limb and the patients are involved, we need an objective scale that indicates the type of patient we are treating. For this purpose, among other scales (e.g. Prevent III and Finnvasc), we have included the categorization of the chronic pluripathological patient adopted by Osakidetza-Servicio Vasco de Salud (Osakidetza-SVS, Basque Country National Health Service) in 2011 based on the good practice model of Kaiser Permanente. Chronic patients are stratified into three levels of intervention depending on the complexity of the case. At the baseline of the Kaiser Permanente pyramid, the healthy members of the population are located for whom prevention, health promotion and risk factor control interventions are a priority. In the first level, where the majority of chronic patients we find concentrated, the interest is focused on promoting self-care. In the second level are chronic patients with the prominence of a particular disease or organ and who can benefit from the "disease management", and, finally, in the highest level of the pyramid are those patients with very complex cases that need integral management. Although they are not the most numerous, these are the ones that consume the most resources [23] (see **Figure 4**).

Other scales used in vascular surgery units are Prevent III and Finnvasc. Prevent III was designed to calculate the amputation-free time after revascularization surgery and consists of a scoring system on various pathologies: dialysis 4 points, tissue loss 3 points, age ≥ 75 years 2 points, hematocrit ≤30% 2 points and coronary disease 1 point. A low risk ≤3, medium risk 4–7 or severe risk ≥8 points is attributed according to the score obtained [24]. Finnvasc score seems to behave better also when predicting the immediate postoperative outcome [25]. The accuracy of these scales is acceptable. They are easy to use and very valuable in clinical practice, especially to help us decide when not to revascularize.

2.1 Population in our study

Based on this background, as part of a doctoral thesis [26], we collected retrospectively our data. The aim of the study was to evaluate the implementation of the WIfI classification mainly on the risk of major amputation and benefit of revascularization at 1 year in a population diagnosed with CLTI and neuro-ischaemic or pure ischaemic wounds and diabetes. Adding up the TASC-II classification to have more information on the arterial status of the limb and the result of applying the Kaiser Permanente pyramid to better profile the type of patient affected.

It is a retrospective and observational study based on episodes of active ulcer in patients with diabetes collected in a prospective database open from the beginning of the care activity related to the creation of the Multidisciplinary Diabetic Foot Unit at Cruces University Hospital.

From February 2011 to June 2012, we treated 122 consecutive patients (151 episodes) with diabetic foot ulcer. The median age was 70 years (SD 11.35). Men are 73.8%. The median HbA1c was 62.8 mmol/mol (7.9%). Hypertension was present in 82% of our population, coronary artery disease in 53%, chronic kidney disease in 38%

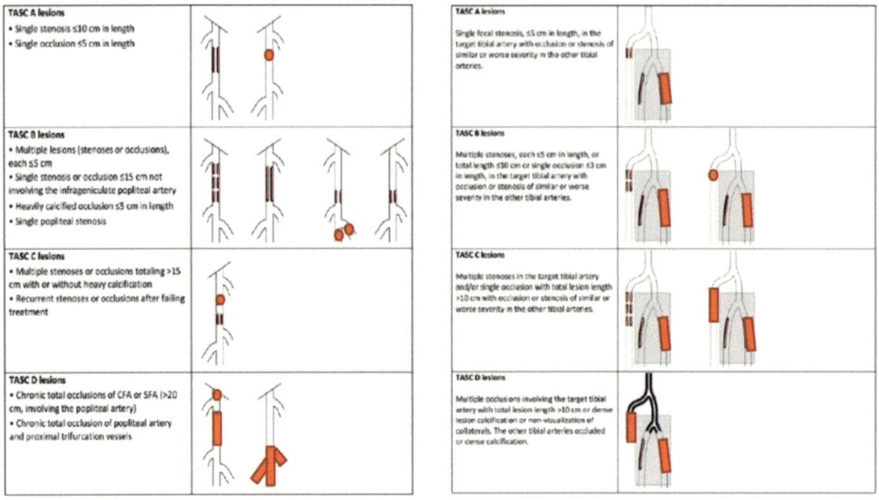

Figure 3.
Modified from TASC-II classification system including below the knee (BTK) lesions [21].

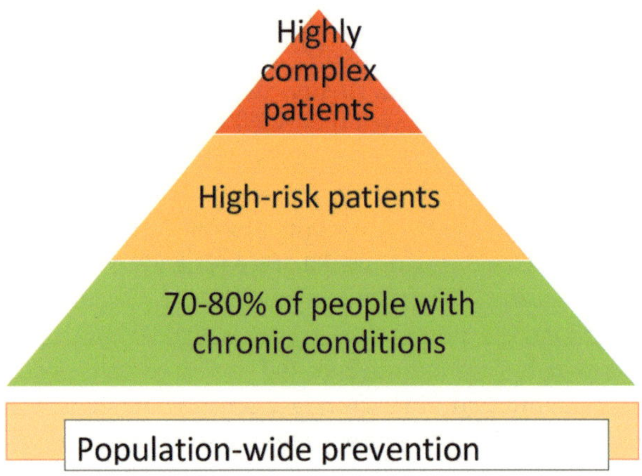

Figure 4.
Adapted from the Kaiser Permanente pyramid model [23].

and 6.0% on dialysis. We retrospectively collected data on 124 (82.11%) ischaemic and neuro-ischaemic ulcers; 27 pure neuropathic (17.89%) were excluded from the study. Therefore 115 ulcers in 93 patients were the final population (see **Figure 5**).

To verify the influence of the different factors on the time to amputation, the survival of the patients or until healing, we make use of Kaplan–Meier tables. A univariate and multivariate Cox regression has also been carried out using a non-automatic stepping method. A level of statistical significance $p < 0.05$ has been considered for all tests. The statistical analysis was carried out with the SPSS program vs. 22.0.

2.2 Our results

In our study 72.6% of patients were revascularized. We follow the "endovascular-first" policy, but whether the intervention was endovascular or open is not specified. We had 18 (14.5%) major amputations at one year. Fourteen of them (78%) were in WIfI stage 4 and 4 (22%) in WIfI stage 3 (see **Table 10**). The positive likelihood ratio (LR) was 1.40 (95% CI = 1.04–1.89); and the negative LR

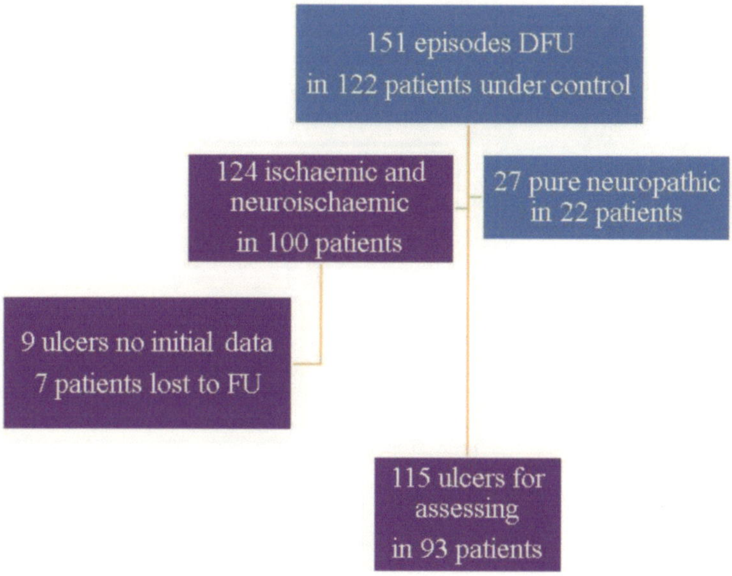

Figure 5.
Population under study [26].

was 0.5 (95% CI = 0.20–1.23). In the negative LR, if a patient was in stage 1, 2 or 3, he/she had double probability for limb salvage than in stage 4.

Regarding the benefit of revascularization, we compared patients classified as high benefit versus those of moderate and low benefit. Those of very low benefit were excluded because the intervention would not really be indicated. The positive LR was 2.08 (95% CI = 1.39–3.13) and negative LR 0.00. Thus, the probability that a patient with a high benefit of being revascularized according to the WIfI scale, if this intervention is performed, saves the limb is 73.1%.

In our study the analysis of the area under the receiver operating characteristic (ROC) curve (AUC) regarding the predictive ability related to amputation risk at 1 year was 0.61 (95% CI = 0.47–0.74) (see **Figure 6**).

2.2.1 Survival function for major amputation

In our population the median time for suffering a major amputation was 4.01 years (95% CI = 3.69–4.31). Patients who had not undergone prior amputation

WIfI amputation risk at 1 year	No	Yes	Total
Very low, Number	5	0	5
%	100.0	0.0	100.0
Low, Number	12	0	12
%	100.0	0.0	100.0
Moderate, Number	30	4	34
%	88.2	11.8	100.0
High, Number	59	14	73
%	80.8	19.2	100.0
Total Number	106	18	124
%	85.5	14.5	100.0

Table 10.
Number of major amputations at 1 year according to WIfI [26].

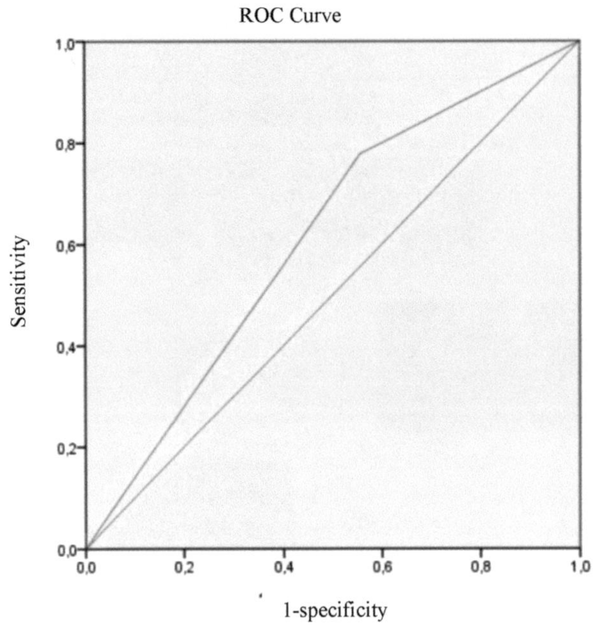

Figure 6.
Area under the ROC curve [26].

and those who had only a minor one take a median of 4.08 years (95% CI = 3.77–4.40) and (95% CI = 3.47–4.69), respectively. Patients who had suffered a previous major amputation were amputated in a median of 1.76 years (95% CI = 0.76–2.77); the difference was statistically significant $p < 0.001$ (see **Figure 7**).

Patients in TASC A, B and C take a median of 4.14 years (95% CI = 3.921–4.367) to suffer a major amputation, whereas patients classified as TASC D took a median of 3.75 years (95% CI = 3.306–4.200). The difference was statistically significant $p = 0.009$ (see **Figure 8**).

We found statistical differences regarding the amputation rate only when WIfI stages 1, 2 and 3 were compared with stage 4. Patients classified according to the WIfI scale as very low, low and moderate risk of being amputated during the first year underwent such amputation in a median of 3.92 years (95% CI = 3.60–4.23). And those classified as high risk presented it in a median of 3.73 years (95% CI = 3.27–4.18), $p = 0.044$ (see **Figure 9**).

Patients with small lesions take a median of 3.90 years to be amputated (95% CI = 3.58–4.23); those with a major lesion took 4.01 years (95% CI = 3.58–4.43) compared to those who had extensive wound that took 1.35 years (95% CI = 0.21–2.48); the difference was statistically significant $p < 0.001$ (see **Figure 10**).

Cox regression multivariate analysis identified previous major amputation, TASC D arterial lesions and extensive ulcer from WIfI (but no global WIfI) as independent risk factors for major amputation (see **Table 11**).

2.2.2 Survival function for survival

We must not forget that we are facing elderly and pluripathological patients. The median survival was 3.42 years (95% CI = 3.08–3.76). Patient's survival was 84% at 1 year, 66% at 3 years and 50% at 5 years. Five years after the diagnosis of CLTI, only half of the population survived regardless of whether the limb was saved or amputated (see **Figure 11**).

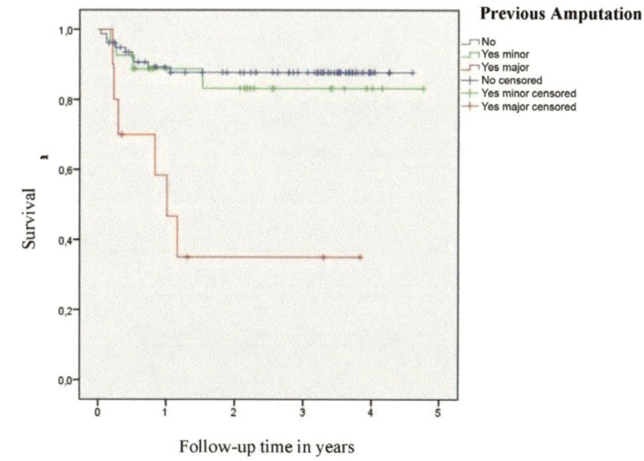

Previous Amputation	Total Number	Events Number	Censored	
			Number	Percentage
No	78	9	69	88.5%
Yes, minor	27	4	23	85.2%
Yes, major	10	6	4	40.0%
Global	115	*19	96	83.5%

*19 Events: One amputation was excluded because it happened after the first year

Figure 7.
Survival function for major amputation according to previous one [26].

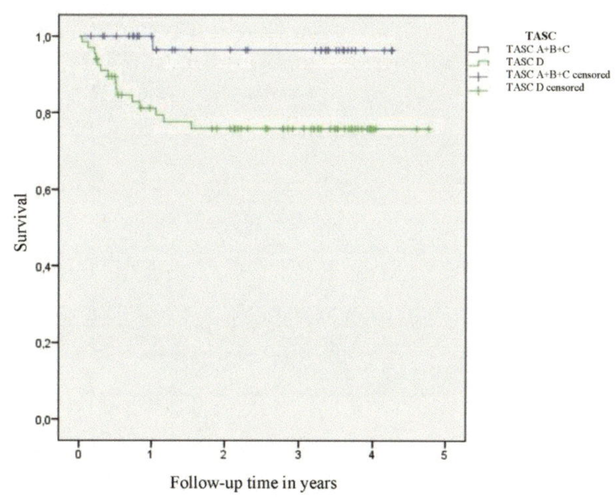

TASC Recoded	Total Number	Events Number	Censored	
			Number	Percentage
TASC A+B+C	39	1	38	97.4%
TASC D	67	15	52	77.6%
Global	106	16	90	84.9%

Figure 8.
Survival function for TASC-II major amputation risk at 1 year comparing a, B and C versus D.

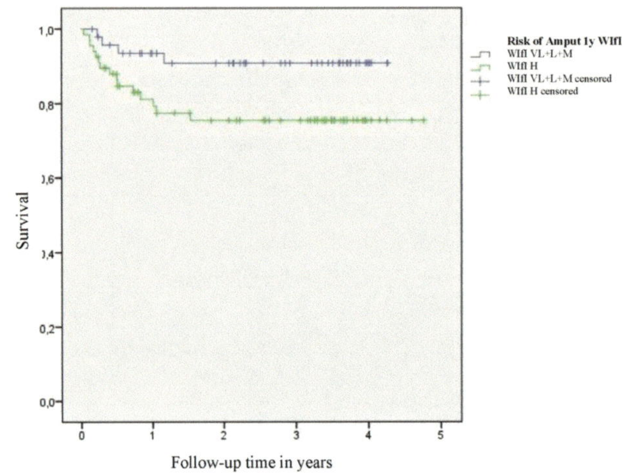

WIfI Recoded	Total Number	Events Number	Censored	
			Number	Percentage
WIfI 1,2,3	48	4	44	91.7%
WIfI 4	67	15	52	77.6%
Global	115	*19	96	83.5%

Figure 9.
Survival function for WIfI major amputation risk at 1 year stages 1, 2 and 3 compared with stage 4 [26].

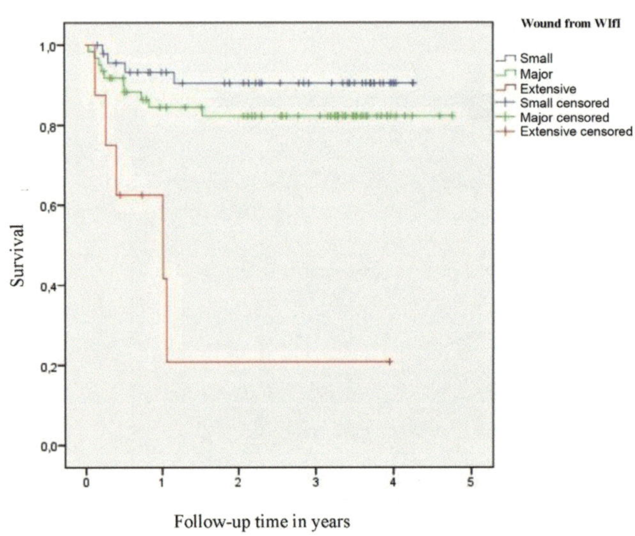

Wound	Total Number	Events Number	Censored	
			Number	Percentage
Small Lesion	46	4	42	91.3%
Major Lesion	61	10	51	83.6%
Extensive Lesion	8	5	3	37.5%
Global	115	19	96	83.5%

Figure 10.
Survival function for major amputation according to wound from WIfI.

			HR 95% CI	
	p-value	**HR**	**Inferior**	**Superior**
No previous amputation (reference)	<0.001			
Yes, minor	0.987	0.987	0.197	4.934
Yes, major	<0.001	20.720	6.013	71.406
TASC D (recoded)	0.003	27.952	3.000	260.452
WIfI extensive lesion (reference)	0.016			
Small lesion	0.194	2.248	0.662	7.632
Major lesion	0.004	11.868	2.184	64.490

Table 11.
Cox regression multivariate analysis for major amputation.

In our study, 51% of patients were in the Kaiser Permanente pyramid highest risk zone. Patients who did not reach the top of the pyramid survive a median of 4.25 years (95% CI = 3.88–4.62), and those who accumulate more pathology survive a median of 3.30 years (95% CI = 2.90–3.70), $p < 0.001$ (see **Figure 12**).

The Cox regression multivariate analysis has shown that only the stratification of the pluripathological patient according to the Kaiser Permanente model is an independent risk factor for death. The most pluripathological patients are classified at the top of the pyramid (red color) and have a risk of dying 8.27 times higher (95% CI = 2.48–27.59).

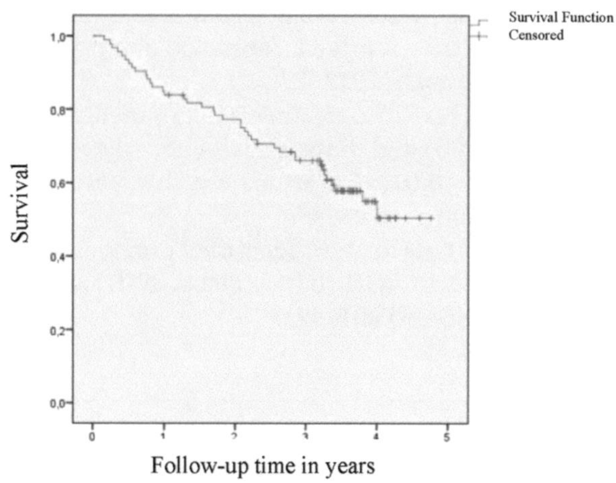

			Censored	
Survival Function	Total Number	Events Number	Number	Percentage
	93	39	54	58.1%

Figure 11.
Patient's survival function [26].

2.2.3 Survival function for wound healing time (WHT)

The median time for ulcer healing, in our study, was 7.65 months (95% CI = 5.723–9.587) which is equal to 230 days.

Previous history of amputation influences wound healing time. Thus, in patients with no past history of amputation, the median WHT was 13.4 months (95% CI = 9.65–17.20); in those with a minor amputation, 15.7 months (95% CI = 10.34–21.20); and in patients with a major one, 34.5 months (95% CI = 23.50–45.55), $p = 0.006$.

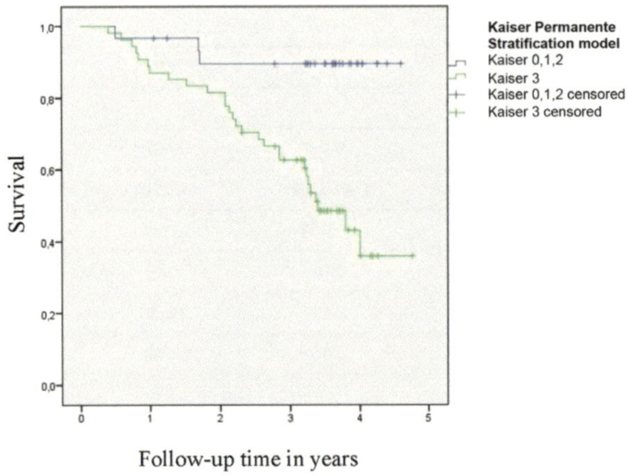

Kaiser Permanent Pyramid	Total N	Events N	Censored	
			N	Percentage
Kaiser 0,1,2	30	3	27	90.0%
Kaiser 3	54	28	26	48.1%
Global	84	31	53	63.1%

Figure 12.
Survival function comparing low and median levels with high level at Kaiser Permanente pyramid [26].

As the arterial lesions become more complex according to TASC-II and more extensive according to WIfI, wound healing time is longer, $p = 0.005$ and $p < 0.001$, respectively. There is more information about WHT in a previous paper published by our group in 2017 [27].

Patients who followed podiatric treatment take a median of 7.5 months in healing (95% CI = 6.14–9.03) and those who did not take a median of 12 months (95% CI = 2.18–22.00), $p = 0.012$. Unfortunately, this factor was only significative at Cox regression univariate analysis.

Cox regression multivariate analysis identified previous amputation, TASC-II classification and wound from WIfI (but no global WIfI) as independent risk factors for wound healing (see **Table 12**).

			HR 95% CI	
	p-value	**HR**	**Inferior**	**Superior**
TASC D (reference)	<0.001			
TASC A	0.001	6.672	2.206	20.181
TASC B	<0.001	5.517	2.208	13.783
TASC C	0.028	1.828	1.068	3.126
Extensive lesion (reference)	0.040			
Small	0.025	9.959	1.336	74.252
Major	0.057	6.985	0.946	51.580
Previous major amputation (reference)	0.008			
No amputation	0.010	13.696	1.868	100.391
Minor amputation	0.044	8.099	1.060	61.874

Table 12.
Cox regression multivariate analysis for wound healing time [26].

2.3 Discussion

Reviewing the van Reijen meta-analysis which compares the best methodological 12 scientific papers published until June 2018 focused on the prognostic value of the WIfI classification in patients with CLTI, only one study included exclusively patients with diabetes, whereas others excluded them.

Regarding treatment, six studies included revascularized patients in different ways, and the other six also included patients with conservative treatment.

The prognostic value of the WIfI classification was studied retrospectively (as in our study) in all but one which implies a certain risk of information bias. Five studies performed a multivariate analysis for the WIfI classification on major amputation, but in four of them, clinical stage or reference was not reported.

The authors recognize that the likelihood of a major amputation after 1 year in patients with CLTI increases with higher clinical WIfI stages, especially in stage 4 in spite of diverging range of patients included (hospitalized/outpatients; requiring hemodialysis or not; invasively or conservative treatment; diabetics/non-diabetics; etc.). This could, partly, explain the statistical heterogeneity that they found. Although the concept of the WIfI classification is well designed, it only considers the status of the affected limb with neither additional information related to vascular anatomy involved nor patients' comorbidities [20] (see **Tables 13** and **14**).

2.4 Conclusions

In conclusion, in our study, we identified a previous amputation, TASC-II classification and wound from WIfI (but no global WIfI) as independent risk factors for major amputation and wound healing time. And, among other comorbidities, only

	% Major amputation >1 year	% AFS >1 year	% Limb salvage >1 year
WIfI I	0	83	95
WIfI II	8	76	92
WIfI III	11	75	91
WIfI IV	38	55	61

Table 13.
Results of van Reijen meta-analysis [20].

	Cull	Zhan	Causey	Beropoulis	Darling	Ward	Vela
Age (years)	70 +/− 11	58 +/− 16	66	77 +/− 15	71 +/− 12	62.8	70 +/− 11
Males %	62	79	62	61	53	—	74
HbA1c %	—	—	—	—	—	—	7.9
DM %	66	93	76	0	77	72	100
Prevent III at high risk	—	—	17%	5.2 +/− 2.4	—	—	—
Kaiser high risk level %	—	—	—	—	—	—	51
Hypertension %	93	86	85	—	84	84	82
CAD %	63	55	47	54	49	—	53
CKD %	—	41	—	37.5	23	—	38
Dialysis %	14	20	23	15.5	18	—	6

Table 14.
Population comparison from some studies included on van Reijen meta-analysis and our study.

the stratification of the pluripathological patient according to the Kaiser Permanente model was recognized as an independent risk factor for death.

Of course, our study has certain limitations: it is retrospective but is based on test and images included in our electronic database. The population is small, and we need to recode some items in order to increase statistical significance. Moreover, our patients are in-hospital, with CLTI and diabetes. But our goal was "the better definition of the population, the better accuracy of the results". Infection was no significant because it was controlled on antibiotics.

In line with other publications, our data support that the WIfI classification system correlates well with clinical outcomes regarding risk of amputation at one year and WHT. However, when adding TASC-II and, in our case, Kaiser Permanente pyramid assessment, the outcome is even more accurate not only for limb salvage but also for patients' survival.

Considering all this information, not only more prospective studies if not a new three-dimensional score capable to predicting the outcome of an individual ulcer paying attention to the better characterization of the population involved should be implemented.

Acknowledgements

First of all, we thank Tania Iglesias-Soria, podiatrist at Multidisciplinary Diabetic Foot Unit (Cruces University Hospital), and Lorea Martínez-Indart, statistical data manager from Biocruces Bizkaia Institute, for their constant support. Second, we also appreciate the Biocruces Bizkaia Institute and Merck Sharp & Dohme de España, S.A. for their technological and economical assistance.

Conflict of interest

The authors declare no conflict of interest.

Author details

Maria Pilar Vela-Orús[1*] and María Sonia Gaztambide-Sáenz[2]

1 Biocruces Bizkaia, Bizkaia Health Research Institute, Vascular Surgeon Consultant, Multidisciplinary Diabetic Foot Unit at Cruces University Hospital, Osakidetza-SVS, Barakaldo-Vizcaya, Spain

2 Biocruces Bizkaia, UPV/EHU, CIBERDEM, CIBERER, Endo-ERN (Project Number 739527), Endocrinologist Consultant and Chief of Department, Multidisciplinary Diabetic Foot Unit at Cruces University Hospital, Osakidetza-SVS, Barakaldo-Vizcaya, Spain

*Address all correspondence to: pilarvelaorus@movistar.es

References

[1] Cavanagh P, Attinger C, Abbas Z, Bal A, Rojas N, Xu ZR. Cost of treating diabetic foot ulcers in five different countries. Diabetes/Metabolism Research and Reviews. 2012;**28** (Suppl. 1):107-111

[2] PRF B, Charlesworth D, De Palma RG, HHG E, Eklöf B, Jamieson CV, et al. The definition of critical ischaemia of a limb. Working party of the international vascular symposium. The British Journal of Surgery. 1982;**69**(Suppl):S2

[3] Aboyans V, Ricco JB, MEL B, Bjorck M, Brodmann M, Cohnert T, et al. Editor's choice - 2017 ESC guidelines on the diagnosis and treatment of peripheral arterial diseases, in collaboration with the European society for vascular surgery (ESVS). European Journal of Vascular and Endovascular Surgery. 2018;**55**:305e68

[4] World Health Organization. WHO Study group on Prevention of Diabetes Mellitus. WHO Technical Report Series; 844. Geneva: WHO; 1994. pp. 63-68

[5] Moulik PK, Mtonga R, Gill GV. Amputation and mortality in new onset diabetic foot ulcers stratified by etiology. Diabetes Care 2003;**26**(2): 491-494

[6] Prompers L, Huijberts M, Apelqvist J, Jude E, Piagessi A, Bakker K et al. High prevalence of ischaemia, infection and serious comorbidity in patients with diabetic foot disease in Europe. Baseline results from the Eurodiale study. Diabetologia. 2007;**50**:18-25

[7] International Consensus on the Diabetic Foot 2015. Prevention and management of foot problems in Diabetes. Guidance documents and recommendations. The international working group on the diabetic foot (IWGDF)/Consultative section of the International Diabetes Federation (IDF) 2007. Actualized in 2011 & 2015

[8] Apelqvist J, Elgzyri T, Larsson J, Löndahl M, Nyberg P, Thöme J. Factors related to outcome of neuroischaemic/ ischaemic foot ulcer in diabetic patients. Journal of Vascular Surgery. 2011;**53**(6): 1582-1588.e2

[9] Elgzyri T, Larsson J, Thörne J, Eriksson KF, Apelqvist J. Outcome of ischaemic foot ulcer in diabetic patients who had no invasive vascular intervention. European Journal of Vascular and Endovascular Surgery. 2013;**46**:110-117

[10] Joslin EP. Menace of diabetic gangrene. The New England Journal of Medicine 1934;**211**:16-20

[11] Edmonds M, Foster A. Reduction of major amputations in the diabetic ischaemic foot: A strategy to "take control" with conservative care as well as revascularization. VASA 2001;**58** (Suppl):6-14

[12] Fitzgerald RH, Mills JL Joseph W and Armstrong DG. The diabetic rapid response acute foot team (DRRAFT): 7 essential skills for targeted limb salvage. Eplasty. 2009;**9**:e15

[13] Rogers LC, Andros G, Caporusso J, Harkless LB, Mills JL, Armstrong DG. Toe and flow: Essential components and structure of the amputation prevention team. Journal of Vascular Surgery. 2010; **52**:23S-27S

[14] Chadwick P, Edmonds M, McCardle J, Armstrong D. International best practice guidelines: Wound Management in Diabetic Foot Ulcers. Wounds International. 2013:1-24. Available from: www.woundsinternational.com

[15] Monteiro-Soares M, Martins-Mendes D, Vaz-Carneiro A, Sampaio S

and Dinis-Ribeiro M. Classification systems for lower extremity amputation prediction in subjects with active diabetic foot ulcer: A systematic review and meta-analysis. Diabetes/Metabolism Research and Reviews. 2014;**30**(7): 610-622

[16] Monteiro-Soares M, Russell D, Boyko EJ, Jeffcoate W, Mills JL, Morbach S et al on behalf of the International Working Group on Diabetic Foot (IWGDF). IWGDF Guideline on the Classification of Diabetic Foot Ulcers. Part of the 2019 IWGDF Guidelines on the Preventionand Management of Diabetic Foot Disease. Diabetes/Metabolism Research and Reviews. 2020;**36**(S1): e3273

[17] Ince P, Zulfiqarali GA, Lutale JK, Basit A, Ali SM, Farooq Ch et al. Use of the SINBAD classification system and score in comparing outcome of foot ulcer management on three continents. Diabetes Care. 2008;**31**:964-967

[18] Lipsky B, Berendt A, Cornia PB. Infectious Diseases Society of America clinical practice guideline for the diagnosis and treatment of diabetic foot infections. IDSA guidelines. Clinical Infectious Diseases. 2012;**54**(12): 132-173

[19] Mills JL, Conte MS, Armstrong DG, Pomposelli FB, Schanzer A, Sidawy AN et al. The Society for Vascular Surgery Lower Extremity Threatened Limb Classification System: Risk stratification based on wound, ischaemia and foot infection (WIfI). Journal of Vascular Surgery. 2014;**59**:220.e2-234.e2

[20] Van Reijen NS, Ponchant K, Ubbink DT and Koelemay MJW. Editor's choice: The prognostic value of the WIfI classification in patients with chronic limb threatening Ischaemia: A systematic review and meta-analysis. European Journal of Vascular and Endovascular Surgery. 2019;**58**:362-371

[21] Jaff MR, White ChJ, Hiatt WR, Fowkes GR, Dormandy J, Razavi M et al. An update on methods for revascularization and expansion of the TASC lesion classification to include below-the-knee arteries: A supplement to the inter-society consensus for the management of peripheral arterial disease (TASC II) Journal of Endovascular Therapy. 2015;**22**:663-667

[22] Hae Won J, Young-Guk K, Sung-Jin H, Chul-Min A, Jung-Sun K, Byeong-Keuk K et al. Editor's choice-impact of endovascular pedal artery revascularization on wound healing in patients with critical limb ischaemia. European Journal of Vascular and Endovascular Surgery. 2019;**58**: 854-863

[23] Feachem RGA, Sekhri NK, White KL. Getting more for their dollar: A comparison of the NHS with California's Kaiser Permanente. BMJ Clinical Research. 2003;**324**(7330):135-141

[24] Schanzer A, Goodney PP, Li Y, Eslami M, Cronenwett J, Messina L et al. Validation of the PIII CLI score for the prediction of amputation-free survival in patients undergoing infrainguinal autogenous vein bypass for critical limb ischaemia. Journal of Vascular Surgery. 2009;**50**(4):769-775

[25] Arvela E, Söderström M, Korhonen M, Halmesmäki K, Albäck A, Lepäntalo M et al. Finnvasc score and modified prevent III score predict long-term outcome after infrainguinal surgical and endovascular revascularization for critical limb ischaemia. Journal of Vascular Surgery. November 2010;**52**(5):1218-1225

[26] Vela-Orús MP [Directed by Gaztambide-Sáenz MS]. Isquemia crítica en pacientes con diabetes. ¿Es válida la nueva clasificación WIfI? [Doctoral Thesis]. Bilbao-Vizcaya. Spain: Euskal Herriko Unibertsitatea/

Universidad del Pais Vasco EHU/UPV; 2016

[27] Vela-Orús MP, Iglesias-Soria T, Martínez-Indart L, Arana-Arri E and Gaztambide-Sáenz S. Evaluation of the WIfI classification system in older patients with diabetes. Wounds International. 2017;**8**(4):23-27

Chapter 9

Diabetic Foot Ulcer: An Easy and Comprehensive Approach

Imran Ali Shaikh, Naila Masood Sddiqui and Javeria Hameed Shaikh

Abstract

Foot problems are commonly involved in diabetes, and the most common presentation of diabetes is an ulcer. Diabetic foot ulcer is a complex problem caused by reduced blood supply, nerve damage, or infection. But unfortunately in most of cases, these three factors have played a role for impairment of diabetic feet. Sometimes nerve damage or neuropathy is an initial insult, and multiple times ischemia is the leading factor for ulcer formation. After certain period, infection finally supervenes and makes a sterile ulcer to infected leads to loss of limb or foot. This becomes more complicated because of less pronounced ischemic symptoms in diabetic than non-diabetics. Furthermore, the healing of a neuroischemic ulcer is slowed down by microvascular dysfunction. Therefore, some ulcers can get better by revascularization, but pure ischemic ulcers rarely respond to revascularization. Many guidelines have largely ignored these specific demands related to ulcerated neuroischemic diabetic feet. Any diabetic foot ulcer should always be considered to have vascular impairment unless otherwise proven. This chapter highlights the best way to diagnose and treat these patients with diabetic foot ulcer. Most of the studies dealing with neuroischemic diabetic feet are not comparable in terms of patient populations, interventions, or outcomes. Therefore, there is an urgent need for a paradigm shift in diabetic foot care, that is, a new approach and classification of diabetics with foot ulcer in regard to clinical practice and research.

Keywords: diabetic, ulcer, Hyderabad, diabetic foot, diabetic foot ulcer, revascularization

1. Introduction

Diabetic foot ulcer is a late and disfiguring complication, which leads to higher risk of amputation of any part of the foot or leg. Therefore diabetic foot disease has major medical, economic, and social consequences. It is very important to treat it with proper protocol to save patients from fatal and disabling complications.

The complexity is to understand the main insult which can be diabetic peripheral arterial disease, neuropathy, or infection. The healing process is also halted due to impaired collagen synthesis. Vascular disease varies from arteritis, occlusion, and large vessel atherosclerosis.

The diabetic foot ulcer is a cave of infection, severe vessel ischemia, and multiple painless traumas. Factors that exacerbate the problem are advanced age, duration of the diabetes, and control of diabetes.

 IntechOpen

Diabetic foot ulcers are classified in many ways, but many systems of classification are complex to interpret. Hence, particular attention to feet care should be a central focus in educating and managing patients with diabetes to ensure that ulcer is either prevented or noticed early enough.

2. Classification and epidemiology of diabetes and foot ulcer

Persistent elevation of blood sugar is associated with major metabolic abnormalities in diabetic patients and damages to various organs and systems, leading to life-threatening complications, which can be overt like major cardiovascular events and cerebrovascular accidents or covert such as retinopathy or nephropathy.

Diabetes mellitus is broadly classified into four types by etiology and clinical presentation, type 1 diabetes, type 2 diabetes, gestational diabetes (GDM), and other less common types of diabetes, which include monogenic diabetes and secondary diabetes.

1. Type 1 diabetes, which involves autoimmune beta-cell destruction, leads to absolute insulin deficiency.

   In the past decade, there was a 21% increase in the number of type 1 diabetes in the USA [1], and the prevalence is increasing at a rate of 3% per year globally [2]. Another study reported that the annual increase was 2% in type 1 diabetes and 5% for type 2 diabetes [3].

   There is no gender variation in type 1 diabetes [4], and type 1 diabetes reduce life expectancy by 13 years as per data reported [5]. Approximately 15% of adults to diagnosed with type 2 diabetes have actually latent autoimmune diabetes of adults, which are a variant of type 1 diabetes [6].

2. Type 2 diabetes (steady loss of beta-cell insulin secretion or insulin resistance).

3. Gestational diabetes mellitus (GDM) (diabetes diagnosed in the second or third trimester of pregnancy).

4. Specific types of diabetes due to other causes:

   - maturity-onset diabetes of the young [MODY] or neonatal diabetes;
   - diseases of the pancreas, for example, cystic fibrosis and chronic pancreatitis; and
   - drug- or chemical-induced diabetes.

Nearly 463 million adults (20–79 years of age) are living with diabetes; by 2045, this will rise to 700 million. The proportion of people with type 2 diabetes is increasing in most countries, and 79% of adults with diabetes are living in low- and middle-income countries. The greatest number of people with diabetes is between 40 and 59 years of age.

In past year, subcontinents were affected enormously. It was estimated that nearly 20 million adults in Pakistan were diabetics, putting them at risk for major or minor complications, and approximately 8 million are still undiagnosed [7].

There are many contributing risk factors for type 2 diabetes: poor socioeconomic status, reduced literacy in 41%, low occupation in 31%, and less income in 40% [8].

More than 15% of diabetic people during their lives experience foot ulcers [6]. These ulcers account for more than 80% of nontraumatic lower limb amputations [9]. The burden of foot ulcer in diabetes varies from 3% in Oceania to 13% in North America, Canada (14.8%), Asia 5.5%, and Europe 5.1% [10].

The annual incidence of diabetic foot ulcer or necrosis in diabetic patients is known to be about 2–5%, and the lifetime risk ranges from 15 to 20% [11].

3. Risk factors for diabetic foot ulcer

Males are affected more than females, and it is more common in **the elderly** above 60 years of age. Several studies have reported **racial predisposition.** One author has evaluated that the increased risk of amputation in African blacks was 2- to 3-fold higher than that in whites [12].

The diabetic foot ulcer is seen in **lower socioeconomic** class (78.2%) [13]. **Smoking** aggravates macrovascular complications including peripheral arterial disease.

It has been observed that 47% of patients who had previous ulceration **walked barefooted** within the house and 17% walked barefooted outside [14]. **Neuropathy** was involved in more than half of diabetic foot ulcers [15], while **peripheral vascular disease** accounts for about 15% alone and 35% in conjunction with neuropathy. The **unequilibrated distribution of pressure** in the foot during walking exposes pressure bearing points to ulceration [16]. The **previous foot ulcers** have tendency to develop recurrent diabetic foot ulcers.

Previous amputation is undoubtedly a big risk factor in 50% of the diabetic foot ulcers. **Inappropriate footwears** produce foot ulcer frequently in diabetes. **Poor vision** contributes due to diabetic retinopathy with the patient unable to properly identify injurious objects. **Minor or major trauma to foot** could be an origin of a chronic ulcer or wound.

4. Pathogenesis of diabetic foot ulcer

It is a worst combination of neuropathy and ischemia. It becomes more complicated by infection. This process leads to impaired wound healing, decreased cell growth factor response, reduced tissue perfusion, and decreased local angiogenesis.

The precise pattern of diabetic neuropathy is not yet completely understood. More evidence has identified the polyol pathway as a major factor in diabetic neuropathy, which leads to oxidative injury. It becomes more complicated when combined with osmotic cell-induced nerve damage, which triggers nerve cell edema. More than half of foot ulcers were caused by neuropathy [17].

Multiple neuropathies are involved in diabetic foot ulcer, which cause impaired pain sensation and impaired temperature sensation. Sensory diabetic neuropathy increases incidence of ulcer at foot approximately sevenfold, compared to diabetic patients without sensory neuropathy [18].

Finally ulcer appeared which may become chronic and combined to atrophy of foot muscles, flexion extension imbalance and also impaired equilibrium. Progressively, repeated pressure at focal points within the foot leads to ulceration. Furthermore, there is reduced sweating and dryness of the skin predisposing to cracks, which become potential sites for frequent ulceration and portals for bacterial entry.

Peripheral arterial disease is a macrovascular complication and an essential contributor to diabetic foot. The endothelial dysregulation that occurs in diabetes leads to reduced production of nitrous oxide (NO), which is a dependable vasodilator and regulates smooth muscle proliferation and leucocyte adhesion, resulting in atherosclerosis and vascular narrowing and ischemia.

The limb or foot ischemia can happen even in the presence of palpable pedal pulses [19].

Also, hyperglycemia promotes increased levels of fibrinogen and plasminogen activator inhibitor which impairs fibrinolysis [20]. These and other abnormalities promote platelet adhesion and thrombosis. In addition, the formation of advanced glycation end products which are compounds formed by the nonenzymatic reaction between sugars and proteins leads to cross linking of molecules in the extracellular matrix of the basement membrane. This alters the structure of the vessels and promotes stiffness [21]. There is also an increased expression of growth factors and adhesion molecules, e.g., intracellular adhesion molecule 1 and vascular endothelial growth factor [22]. Dyslipidemia also contributes to atherosclerosis. In fact, a 1% increase in HbA1C is related to 25–28% of relative risk of peripheral arterial disease [23–26].

Wound healing is defective in diabetes partly due to deficient angiogenesis. It has been noticed that abnormal excessive and inadequate angiogenesis occurs with diabetic complications, delayed closure time, and impaired tissue remodeling [27]. The inadequate mobilization of bone marrow-derived endothelial progenitor cells (EPCs) to the site of injury is another possible mechanism of impaired healing. These cells respond to ischemia and populate the injury site where they form new vessels [28].

About 60% of diabetic foot ulcers have been infected which could be superficial, deep, or more complex such as osteomyelitis [29]. Although typical signs and symptoms could be absent, severe infection could present with systemic symptoms, e.g., fever, chills, and tachycardia. The Infectious Diseases Society of America (IDSA) criteria for severe diabetic foot infection are temperature of >100°F, tachycardia, tachypnea or respiratory alkalosis, leukocytosis, or leucopenia [30]. The commonly isolated organisms are *Staphylococcus aureus*, *S. epidermidis*, and *Streptococcus* species. Methicillin-resistant *S. aureus* (MRSA) complicates 32% of infections, and it is associated with treatment failure. Among anaerobes, *Peptostreptococcus magnus* and *Bacteroides fragilis* have been isolated. The majority of cases are polymicrobial. *S. aureus*, Group B *Streptococcus*, and gram-negative *Bacilli* are associated with limb-threatening infections [31].

5. Classification of diabetic foot ulcer

Wagner classification system: This system focused on physical characteristics of ulcer, depth, and the presence of osteomyelitis or gangrene (0–5) [32].

SINBAD *f* assesses site, ischemia, neuropathy, bacterial infection, and depth and uses a scoring system 0–6. It has been focused on clinical and gross pathological changes of ulcer.

PEDIS classification: This system was designed by the International Working Group on the Diabetic Foot and uses the same five components of S(AD) SAD: perfusion, extent, depth, infection, and sensation. It does not include ulcer location [33].

DEPA classification: This system looks at four aspects of ulcers: depth, extent of bacterial colonization, phase of healing, and associated etiology. Each category is scored from 1 to 3 according to severity.

University of Texas *f* has been proven effective at predicting lower extremity amputation when combined with Wagner classification, and it comprises four grades, A to D, and four stages, 1–4 [34].

Kobe's Classification focused on neuropathy, infection and vasculopathy: Type 1, mainly peripheral neuropathy (PN); type 2, mainly peripheral arterial disease (PAD); type 3, mainly infection; and type 4: all three combined, neuropathy, peripheral arterial disease with infection [35].

SAD stands for sepsis, arteriopathy, and denervation system. The major drawback of this classification is that it is potentially complex and is primarily intended for selecting population for prospective research [36].

Diabetic Ulcer Severity Score (DUSS)

The Diabetic Ulcer Severity Score (DUSS) is based on the categorization of wounds into specific severity subgroups for a comparison of outcomes. Assessment using the DUSS system includes the presence of pedal pulses, the ability to probe to the bone within the ulcer, and ulcer quantity and location. The sum of points determines severity, with the score ranging from 0 to 4.

6. Approach to diabetic foot ulcer

Feature	Neuropathic	Ischemic	Neuroischemic
Sensation	Sensory loss	Pain	Degree of sensory loss
Callus/necrosis	Callus present	Necrosis common	Minimal callus; prone to necrosis
Wound bed	Pink and granulating, surrounded by callus	Pale and sloughy with poor granulation	Poor granulation
Foot temperature and pulses	Warm with bounding	Cool with absent pulses	Cool with absent pulses
Other	Dry skin and fissuring	Delayed healing	Risk of infection
Typical location	Weight-bearing areas of the foot, such as metatarsal heads, the heel, and over the dorsum of clawed toes	Nail edges and between the toes and lateral borders of the foot	Margins of the foot and toes
Prevalence	35%	15%	50%

7. Assessment of risk

Risk category 0 [37]	Risk category 1	Risk category 2	Risk category 3
Norma plantar sensation	Loss of plantar sensation	Loss of plantar sensation or poor circulation or foot deformity or onychomycosis	History of ulceration, neuropathic fracture, or amputation
Low risk	Moderate risk	High risk	Very high risk

8. Investigations

- CBC
- Renal function tests
- CRP and ESR

- Blood sugar levels
- HbA1C
- Blood culture and sensitivity
- X-ray of the foot [38]
- MRI of the foot
- PET scan in osteomyelitis [39]

Ankle brachial index: in normal subjects, the ankle systolic pressure is higher than the brachial systolic pressure. The normal ABI > 1; in the presence of ischemia, it is <0.9. Absent or feeble pulses, with ABI < 0.9, confirm ischemia [40].

Transcutaneous oxygen tension method TcPO2 less than 20 mmHg has been associated with early wound healing failure [41].

- Ultrasound Doppler vascular studies
- CT angiogram

9. Diabetic foot examination

Sensory examination	Vascular examination	Deformity	Ulcer examination
Vibratory perception: 128 Hz tuning fork or electronic tuning fork	Pedal pulses: dorsalis pedis, posterior tibial, perforating peroneal	Bunions, hammertoes, bone spurs, plantarflexed metatarsals, pes cavus foot type	Area, toe, metatarsal forefoot, lateral, medial
Achilles reflex	Erythema or cyanosis	Hallux limitus, Achilles/ gastro equinus, overpronation	Ischemic or neuropathic or mixed
Monofilament test 10 point touch [42]	Intermittent claudication score	Rocker bottom appearance	Small <10 cm, moderate 11–40 cm, severe >40 cm
Vibration perception threshold (VPT)	Temperature comparison between feet	Prior amputation	Cool with absent pulses
Temperature sensation	Dry skin and fissuring	Gait evaluation	Depth; probe test
Pain sensation	Vascular Doppler ultrasonography	Foot drop, atrophy, necrobiosis lipoidica diabeticorum	Healing or nonhealing (inflammatory granulating epithelialization)

10. Treatment

Treating diabetic foot ulcer is an art and involves multiple specialties. The essential team members are physicians, chiropodist, orthopedics, radiologist, and vascular surgeon. The focus would be ensuring targeted HbA1c, revascularization, wound healing with or without debridement, shading of excessive load over foot or limb, and limiting infection by antibiotics and assessment of complications. Focus on the patient's education and nutrition is very important in reducing recurrence of diabetic foot ulcer.

10.1 Offloading

It means reduction, redistribution, or sharing pressures over the ulcer area. It is a well-known fact that offloading is one of the cornerstones of successful diabetic foot ulceration management and prevention. The aim is to reduce the plantar pressure by redistributing it to a larger area, to avoid shear and friction, and to accommodate the deformities [43].

For diabetic foot ulcer, a proper cast is necessary; for example, nonremovable cast devices are the most clinically effective for neuropathic forefoot and mid-foot ulceration. The aim is to immobilize the foot and ankle within the cast, which significantly reduces shear force.

The total contact cast is a below-knee cast that encroaches the lower limb, encasing the whole foot. It is the main cast for mid- and forefoot lesions and for neuropathic noninfected plantar ulcers. Healing was reported in almost 100% cases of ulcers within 5–8 weeks. For non-cast offloading devices, half shoes are designed to offload either the fore or rear foot. We can decide by giving examples below about casting devices:

Rear foot
For weight-bearing:
Crutches with or without a below-knee cast and a half shoe.
For non-weight-bearing:
Leg trough, pressure-relieving mattress and flexible heel cast or pillows.

Mid-foot
Total contact cast, below-knee cast, or fiberglass boot. Felt padding can be shaped to cover the sole of the foot with a cavity at the ulcer site.

Forefoot
Half shoe; leg- or boot-type cast is the most effective method for offloading; sandals with a foam-filled sink in the sole unit located over the ulcer site may also be useful.

Toe
Cut a hole in the part of the shoe overlying the ulcer site to remove the whole toe from shoe.

A recent systematic review has found nonremovable offloading devices like total contact cast to be more effective for ulcer healing than removable offloading devices [44].

11. Control of foot infection

While most DFIs are relatively superficial at presentation, microorganisms can spread contiguously to subcutaneous tissues, including fascia, tendons, muscle, joints, and bones [45, 46].

First-generation cephalosporin, clindamycin, fluoroquinolone, linezolid.

Moderate infection without systemic involvement.

Ticarcillin/clavulanate, piperacillin/tazobactam; second- or third-generation cephalosporin.

Third-generation cephalosporin, impinemen.
Ugly ulcer with systemic signs.
Ticarcillin/clavulanate, piperacillin/tazobactam; + ceftazidime, flucloxacillin + cipro, carbapenem.
Ischemic limb/necrosis/gas forming.
Ticarcillin/clavulanate, piperacillin/tazobactam or carbapenem; second–/third-generation cephalosporin + clindamycin or metronidazole.

12. Control of ischemia

Revascularization surgery: Patients with peripheral ischemia who have significant functional disability should undergo surgical revascularization if medical management fails. This may decrease the amputation risk in patients with ischemic DFUs.

The procedures include open (bypass grafting or endarterectomy) or endovascular techniques (angioplasty with or without stent) [47].

Extracorporeal shock wave therapy acts by increasing angiogenesis and blood supply and cellular proliferation and thus hastening wound healing.

Low-energy lasers have also been used as an adjunctive therapy for DFUs [48].

13. Wound debridement

Ulcers heal more quickly if the surface is clean; physicians must debride impediments to healing, such as necrotic tissue and bacteria. The popular strategy is to do sharp debridement. So removal of necrotic tissue often extends beyond the ulcer bed, and some authorities have recommended to debride deeper tissues also.

Other strategy is to convert bad ulcer to fresh ulcer by excise the already an ulcer, underlying bony prominences. Good results have been reported with this approach [49].

Many other strategies of debridement include physical debridement using wet-to-dry dressing, enzymatic debridement using enzymes like collagenase and papain as ointment preparations, autolytic debridement with the use of moisture-retaining dressings, and biological debridement with the use of larvae of common green bottle fly [50].

14. Wound dressings

Dressings can provide a warm, moist environment required for healing after debridement. Common problems associated with some of these dressings have been dehydration of the ulcer bed, saturation with exudate, and/or the failure to properly apply antibiotics and growth factors needed to promote angiogenesis and granulation tissue. Non-medicated dressings include paraffin gauze, while medicated include Xeroform [51].

Dressing materials include saline-moistened gauze dressings (wet-to-dry), moisture-retaining and antiseptic dressings, silver dressings, and cadexomer.

Chemically treated honey can be used alone or in combination with sterile dressings [52].

In terms of ulcer healing, a meta-analysis of trials in which people with neuropathic foot ulcers received good wound care reported that 24% of ulcers attained complete healing by 12 weeks and 31% by 20 weeks.

In highly exuding ulcers, dressing is essential in managing the high volume of exudate, achieving moisture balance and preventing peri-wound soft tissue damage. The frequency of wound dressing change is important in achieving these goals.

Superabsorbent dressings are designed to absorb high volumes of wound exudate and to hold and lock the fluid into the structure of the dressing, which may reduce the need for frequent dressing changes.

In a wound with low exudate levels, which contains slough, dressings should be selected with the aim of increasing wound moisture to aid autolysis and achieve moisture balance. In the case of black, dry, and necrotic toes due to ischemia, the primary goal is to keep the toe dry, prevent infection, and protect adjoining or adjacent issues.

15. Nutrition and diabetic foot ulcer

As the other factors are important for proper care of diabetic foot ulcer, nutrition has a pivotal role in healing, prevention of recurrence, and fair outcome. Unfortunately, it is a least considered part of diabetic foot ulcer management.

Imran et al. have shown that BMI was significantly associated with severity of ulcer; BMI of 29 was associated with grade 1 ulcer and low BMI of 23 with grade 5 foot ulcer. Over Mini nutritional assessment scale, a score less than 23.5 was associated with advanced foot ulcers, score < 17 was associated with significant p value <0.03, and score in between 17 and 23.5 was associated with p value of 0.05 [53].

16. Charcot arthropathy

Charcot neuroarthropathy, or Charcot foot, is a complication of diabetes mellitus where there is progressive degeneration of the joints. It commonly affects the middle of the foot, hindfoot joints, the ankle, and forefoot joints, and it is believed to result from inflammation in the tissues. The prevalence of Charcot neuroarthropathy is approximately 13% with diabetes [54].

Charcot neuroarthropathy could result in ulceration and infection which can lead to amputation of the limb. Early recognition and intervention is imperative to avoid the rapid progression toward permanent foot deformity, ulceration, and the possibility of limb loss. Once it has started, ongoing inflammation leads to bone deformities.

The acute Charcot arthropathy results in bony reabsorption and multiple spontaneous fractures. Charcot joint changes can be classified into stages.

0 (prodromal): Elevated temperature, with or without foot edema and bounding pulses. The X-ray of foot is less helpful.

1 Developmental, acute: An acute destructive period that is induced by minor trauma resulting in fragmentation of bone and joint dislocation and subluxation. This stage should be verified by a physician early; otherwise, misdiagnosis will lead to permanent deformities.

2 Subacute: The patient presents with decreased edema and healing of fractures.

3 Chronic: Healing, deformity and remodeling of bones seen on xary.

The acute phase is often misdiagnosed and can lead to permanent foot deformity and ulceration, thus increasing the risk of lower extremity amputation [55].

There are three types of Charcot foot classification: clinical, anatomical, and radiological. In clinical practice, Charcot foot can be classified into the acute and chronic stages [56].

The best way to deal with this stage is offloading of the foot, avoid weight-bearing, prevention of aim of chronic deformities. The pain must be reduced managed and assessment of disease activity by physical signs, X-rays or C reactive protein.

The surgery is indicated for correction of deformities. One researcher has been followed up 100 patients for a median of 3.8 years after conservative treatment for Charcot foot [27] and noted amputations in 2.7% and ulcer recurrence in 49%, but some of them have been prevented by earlier surgical intervention [57].

17. Conclusion

Diabetic foot ulcer contributes to be a major cause for morbidity in patients despite of multiple, advanced, and suitable interventions at different levels. This problem could be addressed and managed by encouraging the patient's education, especially to foot care.

Patients should be motivated to care better for themselves by getting involved in learning programs, which highlight the risk factors and consequences of diabetic foot. These patients should be taught in the simple way to examine an ulcer and assess modified risk factors. The synthesis of national and local guidelines on diabetic foot care should be a priority, and the adherence to such guidelines has to be monitored by concerned organizations.

Author details

Imran Ali Shaikh[1]*, Naila Masood Sddiqui[1] and Javeria Hameed Shaikh[2]

1 Department of Medicine, Liaquat University of Medical and Health Sciences, Jamshoro Sindh, Pakistan

2 Department of Physiology, Liaquat University of Medical and Health Sciences, Jamshoro Sindh, Pakistan

*Address all correspondence to: imran2naila@yahoo.com

References

[1] Dabelea D, Mayer-Davis EJ, Saydah S, et al. Prevalence of type 1 and type 2 diabetes among children and adolescents from 2001 to 2009. JAMA. 2014;**311**:1778-1786

[2] Cho NH, Whiting D, Forouhi N, et al. IDF Diabetes Atlas. Diabetes in Children. 2015;**7**:14-16

[3] Mayer-Davis E, Lawrence JM, Dabelea D, et al. Incidence trends of Type 1 and Type 2 diabetes among youths. NEJM. 2017;**376**:1419-1429

[4] Maahs DM, West NA, Lawrence JM, et al. Epidemiology of type 1 diabetes. Endocrinology and Metabolism Clinics of North America. 2010;**39**:481-497

[5] Livingstone SJ, Levin D, Looker HC, et al. Estimated life expectancy in a Scottish cohort with type 1 diabetes, 2008-2010. JAMA. 2015;**313**:37-44

[6] Stenström G, Gottsäter A, Bakhtadze E, et al. Latent autoimmune diabetes in adults: Definition, prevalence, β-cell function, and treatment. Diabetes. 2005;**54**:S68

[7] Cho NH. Estimates of diabetes for projections to 2030 and 2045. IDF Diabetes Atlas. 2019:9-10. Available from: http://doi.org/10.1016/j.diabetes.2019.107843

[8] Allebeck P, Hallqvist J, Moradi T, et al. Type 2 diabetes incidence and socio-economic position: A systematic review and meta-analysis. International Journal of Epidemiology. 2011;**40**:804-818

[9] Trautner C, Haastert B, et al. Incidence of lower limb amputations and diabetes. Diabetes Care. 1996;**9**:1006-1009

[10] Zhang P, Lu J, Jing Y, Tang S, Zhu D, et al. Global epidemiology of diabetic foot ulceration: A systematic review and meta-analysis. Annals of Medicine. 2017;**49**:106-116

[11] Khanolkar MP, Bain SC, Stephens JW. The diabetic foot. QJM. 2008;**101**(9):685-695

[12] Leggetter S, Fuller JH, et al. Ethnicity and risk of diabetes-related lower extremity amputation. Archives of Internal Medicine. 2002;**162**(1):73-78

[13] Adeleye JO. Diabetic foot disease: The perspective of a Nigerian tertiary health care center. Practical Diabetes International. 2005;**22**(6):211-214

[14] Gulliford MC, Mahabir D. Diabetic foot disease and foot care in a Caribbean community. Diabetes Research and Clinical Practice. 2002;**56**(1):35-40

[15] Dyck PJ, Davies JL, Wilson DM, Service FJ, et al. Risk factors for severity of diabetic polyneuropathy: Intensive longitudinal assessment of the Rochester Diabetic Neuropathy Study Cohort. Diabetes Care. 1999;**22**:1479-1486

[16] Kruse I, Endelman S. Evaluation and treatment of diabetic foot ulcers. Clinical Diabetes. 2006;**24**:91-93

[17] Clayton W, Elcasy TA. A review of the pathophysiology, classification, and treatment of foot ulcers in diabetic patients. Clinical Diabetes. 2009;**27**:52-58

[18] Wild S, Roglic G, Green A, Sicree R, King H. Global prevalence of diabetes: Estimates for the year 2000 and projections for 2030. Diabetes Care. 2004;**27**:1047-1053

[19] Armstrong DA. Lavery LADiabetic foot ulcers: Prevention, diagnosis and classification. American Family Physician. 1998;**57**:1325-1332

[20] Vinik AI, Erbas T, et al. Platelet dysfunction in type 2 diabetes. Diabetes Care. 2001;**24**(8):1476-1485

[21] Cooper ME, Bonnet F, Oldfield M, et al. Mechanism of diabetic vasculopathy: An overview. American Journal of Hypertension. 2001;**14**:475-486

[22] Basta G, Lazzerini G, et al. Advanced glycation end-product activate endothelium signal-transduction receptor RAGE. A mechanism for amplification of inflammatory responses. Circulation. 2002;**105**:816-822

[23] Bucala R, Makita Z, Vega G, et al. Modification of low density lipoprotein by advanced glycation end-products contribute to the dyslipidemia of diabetes and renal insufficiency. Protocol for the National Academy of Sciences USA. Medical Science. 1994;**91**:9441-9445

[24] Okonkwo UA, Di Pietro LA. Diabetes and wound angiogenesis. International Journal of Molecular Sciences. 2017;**18**(7):1419

[25] Dinh T, Veves A. Microcirculation of the diabetic foot. Current Pharmaceutical Design. 2005;**11**(18):2301-2309

[26] Selvin E, Marinopoulos S, Berkenblit G, Rami T, et al. Meta-analysis: Glycosylated hemoglobin and CVD disease in diabetes mellitus. Annals of Internal Medicine. 2004;**21**: 421-431

[27] Ayuk SM, Abrahamse H, et al. The role of matrix metalloproteinases in diabetic wound healing in relation to photo bio modulation. Journal of Diabetes Research. 2016;**2016**:9. Article ID 289756. Available from: http//dx.doi.org/10.1155/2016/2897656

[28] Brem H, Tomic-Canic M. Cellular and molecular basis of wound healing in diabetes. Journal of Clinical Investigation. 2007;**117**(5):1219-1222

[29] Prompers L, Huijberts M, Apelqvist J, et al. High prevalence of ischemia, infection and serious comorbidity in patients with diabetic foot disease in Europe. Baseline results from the Eurodiale study. Diabetologia. 2007;**50**(1):18-25

[30] Lipsky BA, Anthony R, et al. Infectious Diseases Society of America clinical practice guidelines for the diagnosis and treatment of diabetic foot infections. Clinical Infectious Diseases. 2012;**54**(12):132-173

[31] Gadepalli R, Dhawan B, Sreenivas V, et al. A clinico-microbiological study of diabetic foot ulcers in an Indian tertiary care hospital. Diabetes Care. 2006;**29**:1727-1732

[32] Wagner FW. The dysvascular foot: A system of diagnosis and treatment. Foot & Ankle. 1981;**2**:64-122

[33] Chuan F et al. Reliability and validity of the perfusion, extent, depth, infection and sensation (PEDIS) classification system and score in patients with diabetic foot ulcer. PLoS One. 2015;**10**(4):e0124739

[34] Armstrong D, Lavery LA, Harkless LB. Validation of a diabetic wound classification system: The contribution of depth, infection and ischemia to risk of amputation. Diabetes Care. 1998;**21**(5):855-859

[35] Terashi H, Kitano I, Tsuji Y. Total management of diabetic foot ulcerations: Kobe classification as a new classification of diabetic foot wounds. The Keio Journal of Medicine. 2011;**60**:17-21

[36] Macfarlane RM, Jeffcoate WJ. Classification of diabetic foot ulcers: SAD system. The Diabetic Foot. 1999;**2**(4):123-130

[37] Game F. Classification of diabetic foot ulcers. Diabetes/Metabolism Research and Reviews. 2015;**32**(1):186-194

[38] Rajbhandari SM, Jenkins RC, Davies C, Tesfaye S. Charcot neuroarthropathy in diabetes mellitus. Diabetologia. 2002;**45**:1085-1096

[39] Madan SS, Pai DR. Charcot neuroarthropathy of the foot and ankle. Orthopaedic Surgery. 2013;**5**(2):86-93

[40] Doobay AV, Anand SS. Sensitivity and specificity of the ankle-brachial index to predict future cardiovascular outcomes: A systematic review. Arteriosclerosis, Thrombosis, and Vascular Biology. 2005;**25**:1463-1469

[41] Pecoraro RE, Ahroni JH, Boyko EJ, Stensel VL. Chronology and determinants of tissue repair in diabetic lower-extremity ulcers. Diabetes. 1991;**40**(10):1305-1313

[42] Boyko EJ, Ahroni JH, Cohen V, Nelson KM, Heagerty PJ. Prediction of diabetic foot ulcer occurrence using commonly available clinical information: The Seattle Diabetic Foot Study. Diabetes Care. 2006;**29**:1202-1207

[43] Verity S, Sochocki M, Embil JM, Trepman E. Treatment of Charcot foot and ankle with a prefabricated removable walker brace and custom insole. Foot and Ankle Surgery. 2008;**14**:26-31

[44] Morona JK, Buckley ES, Jones S, Reddin EA, Merlin TL. Comparison of the clinical effectiveness of different off-loading devices for the treatment of neuropathic foot ulcers in patients with diabetes: A systematic review and metaanalysis. Diabetes/Metabolism Research and Reviews. 2013;**29**:183-193

[45] Lipsky BA, Aragón-Sánchez J, Diggle M. IWGDF guidance on the diagnosis and management of foot infections in persons with diabetes. Diabetes/Metabolism Research and Reviews. 2016;**32**(1):45-74

[46] LoGerfo FW, Gibbons GW, Pomposelli FB Jr, Campbell DR, Miller A, et al. Trends in the care of the diabetic foot. Expanded role of arterial reconstruction. Archives of Surgery. 1992;**127**(5):617-621. DOI: 10.1001/archsurg.1992.01420050145019

[47] Albayati MA, Shearman CP. Peripheral arterial disease and bypass surgery in the diabetic lower limb. The Medical Clinics of North America. 2013;**97**:821-834

[48] Schindl A, Schindl M, Schön H, Knobler R, Havelec L, et al. Low intensity laser irradiation improves skin circulation in patients with diabetic microangiopathy. Diabetes Care. 1998;**21**:580-584

[49] Pai DR, Madan SS. Techniques in chronic wound management: Review of the literature and recent concepts. Journal of Novel Physiotherapies. 2013;**3**:22-27

[50] Wong MW, Leung PC, Wong WC. Limb salvage in extensive diabetic foot ulceration—A preliminary clinical study using simple debridement and herbal drinks. Hong Kong Medical Journal. 2001;7:403-407

[51] Wu L, Norman G, Dumville JC, et al. Dressings for treating foot ulcers in people with diabetes: An overview of systematic reviews. Cochrane Database of Systematic Reviews. 2015;**14**(7):CD101471

[52] Shukrimi A, Sulaiman AR, Halim AY, Azril A. A comparative study between honey and povidone iodine as dressing solution for Wagner type II diabetic foot ulcers. The Medical Journal of Malaysia. 2008;**63**:44-46

[53] Shaikh IA, Masood N, Shaikh FA, Shaikh MA. Diabetic foot ulcers; correlation of nutritional status of type 2 diabetic patients of Hyderabad Sindh, Pakistan. The Professional Medical Journal. 2017;**24**(5):707-712

[54] Younis BB, Shahid A, Arshad R, Khurshid S, Masood J. Charcot osteoarthropathy in type 2 diabetes persons presenting to specialist diabetes clinic at a tertiary care hospital. BMC Endocrine Disorders. 2015;**15**:28

[55] Wukich D, Sung W, Wipf S, Armstrong DG. The consequences of complacency: Managing the effects of unrecognized Charcot feet. Diabetic Medicine. 2011;**28**(2):195-198

[56] Rogers LC, Frykberg RG. The charcot foot. Medical Clinics of North America. 2013;**97**(5):847-856

[57] Saltzman CL, Hagy ML, Zimmerman B, et al. How effective is intensive nonoperative initial treatment of patients with diabetes and Charcot arthropathy of the feet? Clinical Orthopaedics and Related Research. 2005;**435**:185-190

Chapter 10

Diagnosis, Treatment, Multidisciplinary Collaborative Therapy and Prevention of Diabetic Foot

Fanna Liu and Lianghong Yin

Abstract

Diabetic foot (DF) is one of the most common complications of diabetes. Diabetic foot is one of the main causes of disability and death of diabetic patients, and it is also a major public health problem that causes a heavy burden on society. Diabetic foot involves a variety of factors including peripheral nerve tissue lesions, ischemic lesions, and reduced body immunity. With the development of medical standards, clinical knowledge and treatment of diabetic foot are constantly improving. Early diagnosis and intervention is the key to reducing the incidence of diabetic foot and improving the cure rate. This chapter will briefly introduce the diagnosis, the treatment, the multidisciplinary collaborative therapy and prevention of diabetic foot.

Keywords: diabetic foot, multidisciplinary collaborative therapy, prevention

1. Introduction

Diabetes Mellitus is a chronic non-communicable epidemic that has become the most important in the world. Diabetic foot (DF) is one of the most common complications of diabetes. The global prevalence of diabetic foot is 6.3%, male are higher than female, and type 2 diabetes is higher than type 1 diabetes. The prevalence of diabetic foot varies greatly from country to country, varying from 1.5 to 16.6% [1]. DF is one of the primary causes of disability and death of diabetic patients, and it is also a major public health problem that causes a heavy burden on society.

It is estimated that there is one amputation of diabetic patients every 20 seconds in the world [2]. According to the statistics of the World Health Organization, about 50% of all non-traumatic amputations are due to diabetic foot amputation [3]. The annual mortality rate of patients with diabetic foot is as high as 11%, and the mortality rate of amputated patients is as high as 22% [4]; many studies have shown that diabetic foot costs are huge, accounting for about one-third of the entire diabetes medical cost. In 2017, the global medical cost of diabetes was as high as 727 billion US dollars, of which China was 110 billion US dollars [5]. In developed countries, diabetic foot occupies 12–15% of diabetes medical and health resources, while in developing countries, up to 40% [6]. One third of the medical cost of diabetes in the United States is used for diabetic foot patients [7].

Diabetic foot is the most common cause of hospitalization, with the characteristics of long hospital time, difficult treatment and high medical cost. According to recent big data from the United States, compared with ambulatory diabetic outpatients, diabetic foot patients are 3.4 times more hospitalized or emergency patients, 2.1 times more referrals to specialists, and 1.9 times more annual visits. Physicians spend more time on diagnosis and treatment; patients with diabetic foot infection (DFI) are directly referred to the emergency department or hospitalized by 6.7 times.

Diabetic foot is one of the main causes of disability and death of diabetic patients, and it is also a major public health problem that causes a heavy burden on society.

Diabetic foot involves a variety of factors including peripheral nerve tissue lesions, ischemic lesions, and reduced body immunity. It can be seen that the diagnosis and treatment of diabetic foot need to involve multiple disciplines and fields. With the development of medical standards, clinical knowledge and treatment of diabetic foot are constantly improving. Early diagnosis and intervention is the key to reducing the incidence of diabetic foot and improving the cure rate.

2. Definition and classification of diabetic foot

2.1 The definition of diabetic foot

The causes of diabetic foot are multifactorial. Diabetic peripheral vascular disease, peripheral neuropathy and infection are the basic causes of diabetic foot, which can exist alone or in combination with other factors.

Diabetic foot is the destruction of the skin and deep tissues of the ankle joint of diabetic patients. It is often complicated by infection and/or arterial occlusive disease of different degrees in the lower extremities. In severe cases, muscle and bone tissues are involved. The World Health Organization has a clear definition of diabetic foot, foot infection, ulcers and deep tissue damage caused by abnormal nerves in the lower extremities and varying degrees of lesions in the surrounding blood vessels.

The following people are prone to diabetic foot: old, living alone, male, with a diabetes course of more than 10 years, a history of paraplegia, uncontrolled high blood sugar, and little knowledge about diabetes, combined with foot mold, deformity, calluses, etc.

2.2 Diabetic foot classification

For a DF patient, a comprehensive systemic condition assessment and a foot assessment are necessary. The foot assessment includes the blood supply of the foot, the size and depth of the ulcer, the condition and severity of ulcer infection. Diabetic foot ulcer classification assessment: cause classification, nature classification, then grading and staging, and finally select the appropriate treatment method according to grading and staging.

At present, the common clinical grading methods of diabetic feet include Wagner Ulcer Classification and University of Texas Diabetic Wound Classification. Wagner Ulcer Classification method is currently the most classic grading method. It is divided into 6 levels according to the depth of skin damage and the presence or absence of gangrene. The advantage of this grading system is that it is easy to use in clinical applications. It can be graded without auxiliary examination tools, and can also reflect the severity of ulcers and gangrene. The disadvantage of this system is that it does not reflect the etiology of the foot and lacks reproducibility and specificity when grading ulcers. In addition, superficial cases with or without ischemia cannot be correctly graded, and ischemia is only mentioned in grades 4 and 5.

2.2.1 The Wagner classification of diabetes

Grade 0, No ulcers in a high-risk foot.
Grade 1: Superficial Diabetic Ulcer.
Grade 2: Ulcer extension Involves ligament, tendon, joint capsule or fascia.
No abscess or Osteomyelitis.
Grade 3: Deep ulcer with abscess or Osteomyelitis.
Grade 4: Gangrene to portion of forefoot.
Grade 5: Extensive gangrene of foot [8].

2.2.2 University of Texas Diabetic Wound Classification

Stages.
Stage A: No infection or ischemia.
Stage B: Infection present.
Stage C: Ischemia present.
Stage D: Infection and ischemia present.
Grading.
Grade 0: Epithelialized wound.
Grade 1: Superficial wound.
Grade 2: Wound penetrates to tendon or capsule.
Grade 3: Wound penetrates to bone or joint [9].

3. Pathogenesis of diabetic foot

3.1 Neuropathy

Peripheral neuropathy is one of the important causes of diabetic foot. Relevant research data shows that patients with diabetes over 25 years have a 50% chance of developing peripheral neuropathy, and diabetic foot patients have the highest proportion of with neuropathy [10]. Studies have confirmed that the occurrence of neuroarthropathy is related to autonomic neuropathy; motor neuropathy can lead to metatarsal deformation in diabetic patients, foot muscle atrophy, and increased plantar pressure. In addition, neuropathy can cause diabetic patients to lose their ability to feel external stimuli and injuries, which is also a high-risk factor in the formation of skin injuries such as burns and abrasions.

3.2 Vascular disease

Vascular disease is another important cause of diabetic foot. Long-term hyperglycemia in diabetic patients can cause lesions such as vascular intima damage and vascular occlusion. When the vascular lesions of the lower extremities occur in diabetic patients, they can lead to ischemia and hypoxia in the lower extremities, especially the feet, so that when they urgently need to increase blood circulation, the blood flow cannot increase accordingly, ulcers or even gangrene will occur. In addition, microcirculation disorders caused by vascular lesions can also lead to neuron dystrophy and aggravate nerve function damage, thereby increasing the incidence of ulcers.

3.3 Infection

Leukocyte dysfunction caused by dysglycemia in diabetic patients can lead to decreased immunity of the patient and prone to infection. Infection is also an important inducer of diabetic foot gangrene, and severe cases may even cause sepsis and be life-threatening. Studies have shown that Gram-positive cocci such as *Staphylococcus aureus* and *Enterococcus faecalis* are the main infections of mild infections, and Gram-negative bacillus infections of Proteus and *Escherichia coli* are the main infections of moderate and severe infections.

3.4 Others

Foot deformity, smoking, obesity, visual impairment, alcoholism, and lack of knowledge about diabetic foot are all closely related to the occurrence of diabetic foot.

4. Treatment of diabetic foot

4.1 Medical treatment of diabetic foot disease

Comprehensive medical treatment is the basis of diabetic foot treatment, including strict control of blood sugar and blood pressure, lipid regulation, anti-infection, improvement of microcirculation, correction of hypoproteinemia, elimination of edema and various adverse factors affecting prognosis, etc.

4.1.1 Basic treatment

The basic treatments of diabetic foot mainly include blood sugar control, improve systemic nutrition, strengthen anti-infective treatment, control blood pressure, blood lipids, improve local circulation and blood oxygen.

4.1.2 Blood sugar control

Diabetes patients due to long-term high blood sugar, glucose and nucleic acid and other macromolecular substances combine to cause damage or abnormal function of vascular endothelial cells, and then the blood vessel coagulation function is disordered, causing thrombosis and microcirculation disorders, and ultimately leading to extremities, especially feet ischemia, hypoxia, metabolic disorders, and even ulcer necrosis [11].

Several studies have confirmed that good blood sugar control can effectively reduce the incidence of microvascular disease. Intensive blood glucose management with the A1C goal of <7% is associated with a reduction of microvascular and neuropathic complications of diabetes, and also can lead to a 25% risk reduction of amputation compared to less intensive glycemic management [12]. One systematic review of 19,234 patients also concluded that enhanced blood glucose control can significantly reduce the risk of amputation in patients with DF.

4.1.3 Blood pressure and blood lipid control

Hypertension is the main risk factor for lower extremity arterial disease. For diabetic patients with hypertension, early control of blood pressure can significantly reduce the occurrence of macrovascular disease. Angiotensin converting enzyme inhibitors are recommended, but other antihypertensive drugs can also be used. Diabetes patients with lower extremity arterial disease are often accompanied by dyslipidemia [13]. On the basis of diet control and exercise lipid-lowering, combined with statin lipid-lowering treatment can help the healing of foot ulcers [14].

4.1.4 Infection control

Diabetic foot infection (DFI) is one of the most important causes of patients' deterioration, amputation and death. However, after proper treatment, most patients can be cured. Therefore, active treatment of DFI is beneficial to patients, society, and economy. Multi-drug resistant bacterial infections often indicate a poor prognosis [15].

Once DFI is established, the severity of DFI must be graded. The classification tool recommends the IWGDF/IDSA infection grading system. Antibiotic treatment of diabetic foot infections cannot replace thorough wound debridement treatment. Thorough and adequate debridement and drainage is the basis of effective anti-infective treatment [16].

Treatment principles: thorough and effective debridement is directly related to wound healing. For different types of wounds, the timing debridement should be accurately grasped; physical debridement is the basis of wound treatment. When physical debridement is not suitable, autolytic debridement, Enzymatic debridement, traditional dressing debridement and maggot debridement and other types of debridement should be considered. Decompression treatment of diabetic foot ulcers should adhere to the principle of individualization and continuity, combined with the condition of infection and lower limb ischemia, patients' wishes and ulcers types.

A prospective study of diabetic foot ulcer patients with co-infection showed that in the first year after infection, 15.1% of patients died and 17.4% of patients had at least part of their lower limbs amputated [17]. Studies have found that 49% of diabetic foot ulcer infections are mixed infections. The main pathogens are *Staphylococcus aureus*, *Pseudomonas aeruginosa*, and Enterobacteriaceae [18]. In addition to timely and reasonable surgical treatment of wounds, it is necessary to select antibiotics against common pathogens and early anti-infective treatment according to experience before obtaining the results of pathogenic examinations, and adjust sensitive antibiotics according to the results of pathogenic examinations. In order to improve the positive rate of culture, it is recommended to carry out pathogenic culture or histological examination of deep tissue scrapes before antibiotic treatment, and avoids the use of swab specimens [19]. The use of antibiotics is not recommended for ulcers without signs of infection, the initial antibiotic treatment plan for foot ulcers with infection is an empirical choice, but requires the cultivation of ulcer tissue microorganisms before the application of antibiotics. If clinical treatment is effective, although microbial culture plus drug sensitivity tests show insensitivity, the original treatment plan is suggested. If the patient is not effective with the empirical plan or the infection progresses, antibiotics need to be replaced according to the culture results; mild infection (skin or subcutaneous tissue) takes 1–2 weeks of treatment; moderate to severe infection 2–3 weeks.

For patients with diabetic foot combined with osteomyelitis, the diagnostic methods include clinical examination, such as probe and bone test (probe to bone test): the method has a sensitivity of 66%, a specificity of 85%, and a positive predictive value 89%. X-ray radiograph is little significance for the diagnosis of osteomyelitis, and repeated radiographs every 2–4 weeks can find bone destruction and increase the detection rate of osteomyelitis, MRI is more sensitive to the diagnosis of osteomyelitis 95%, but less sensitive to osteomyelitis with smaller bones. Bone scan and CT are of little significance for the diagnosis of osteomyelitis, bone biopsy is the gold standard for diagnosis, and histological culture results can guide antibiotic selection.

Treatment methods include: anti-infection alone, anti-infection combined with minor surgery: drainage of pus, removal of infected bone, etc.; amputation (toe) combined with antibiotic treatment. Compared with surgical treatment, antibiotics alone are cheaper to treat osteomyelitis, but about 17% are ineffective. Gram-positive cocci infections are the most common bacteria. Broad-spectrum antibiotics are usually selected, and the course of treatment is 6 weeks to 6 months.

4.2 Local wound management of diabetic foot ulcers

4.2.1 Specialized nursing

Local treatment of the wound surface is essential for the healing of diabetic foot ulcers. If treated properly, it can accelerate the healing of ulcers. The "wet healing theory" and "wound bed preparation theory" are innovative developments in chronic wound specialty care in recent years. Wet healing has the following advantages: regulating the oxygen tension of the wound surface and promoting the formation of capillaries, retaining the content contained in the wound exudate tissue proteolytic enzyme is conducive to the dissolution of necrotic tissue and fibrin, promotes the release of various growth factors, maintains the constant temperature of the wound, facilitates the growth of the tissue, without the formation of scabs, and avoids the mechanical damage of the new granulation tissue, protects the nerve endings of the wound, and reduce pain. The core content of "wound bed preparation" is that the wound surface can be divided into four stages of black, yellow, red, and pink according to the color of the wound base. The black stage and the yellow stage are suggested to use of debridement and the use of antibacterial dressings to remove necrosis, and bacterial load. In the red period, treatment with growth factors such as basic fibroblast growth factor, hydrogel dressing, alginate dressing, etc. can promote the proliferation of granulation tissue of the wound surface and quickly fill the wound defect. The powder phase is mainly to protect the wound surface and promote epithelialization, and perform skin grafting when necessary.

4.2.2 Debridement technology

In terms of debridement technology, in addition to traditional surgical debridement, some new debridement techniques have emerged. Such as autolytic debridement, chemical (protein solubilizing enzyme) debridement, mechanical debridement (including ultrasonic debridement waterjet and wound negative pressure treatment, etc.) and biological (maggot) debridement, etc.. These techniques have their own advantages and disadvantages, so clinicians should master their adaptations and contraindications, choose the most appropriate debridement method for different ulcer conditions, and ensure the maximum therapeutic effect. In addition, the above method is only applicable to neurological ulcers or neurovascular ischemic ulcers. For ischemic ulcers, if the affected limb ischemia is severe, excessive local debridement should be avoided. Vasodilator drugs, intraluminal balloon dilation, stent placement, or vascular bypass surgery and autologous stem cell transplantation can be used to improve limb blood supply. When the blood supply of the affected limb improves, local debridement treatment can be performed to remove excessive keratosis, infected and inactivated tissues.

4.2.3 Dressing

The application of dressings can help promote the healing of ulcers, and the "wound bed preparation theory" can guide the choice of dressings. It is clinically recommended to use hydrogel dressing in the black period to fully soften dry necrotic tissue; the yellow period mainly removes bacterial load, absorbs excessive wound exudate, promotes the growth of granulation, transitions to the red period, alginate dressing, hydraulic adhesive dressings and antimicrobial dressings are suitable choices. The red stage and powder stage are the period of granulation and epithelial growth, and the leakage is reduced, ultra-thin hydrocolloid dressings or biological dressings containing growth factors can be choose.

4.2.4 Growth factors

The wound repair process involves the role of many cytokines, including epidermal growth factor, vascular endothelial growth factor, transforming growth factor -β, fibroblast growth factor and erythropoietin, etc. These cytokines have a promoting effect on the proliferation of fibroblasts and capillaries, the migration, granulation tissue growth and wound epithelialization, which ultimately promotes wound healing in diabetic patients [20]. In terms of promoting the growth of ulcer granulation, there are currently a variety of synthetic growth factors such as platelet-derived growth factor, basic fibroblast growth factor, human epidermal growth factor and transforming growth factor [21, 22]. In addition, APG shows a more obvious advantage in the treatment of refractory skin ulcer sinus tract closure. Survival analysis of sinus tract closure time suggests that the closure rate of APG treatment on the sinus tract is significantly better than standard treatment, suggesting that APG is used to treat refractory diabetic skin. Effective, safe and feasible in ulcers.

4.3 Surgical treatment of diabetic foot disease

For those with severe ischemia and poor medical treatment, surgical methods should be used. The ultimate goal is to reduce the pain caused by ischemia, promote ulcer healing, avoid amputation due to limb necrosis, and improve the quality of life. The surgical treatment of diabetic foot mainly includes percutaneous endovascular interventional therapy, surgical vascular bypass reconstruction, stem cell transplantation and amputation.

For patients who are ineffective for medical treatment and are not suitable for minimally invasive treatment of the vascular cavity, surgical vascular reconstruction surgery is recommended. Surgical treatment includes arterial endarterectomy, artificial blood vessel and/or autovascular bypass. Surgical treatment requires that the patient can tolerate anesthesia and surgical shock.

Percutaneous endovascular interventional treatment includes traditional percutaneous balloon dilatation (PTA), stent implantation, percutaneous intimal circumcision, and Pedal-Plantar Loop technology for small vessel disease of the foot. In recent years, with the invention of new types of balloons and stents (drug-coated balloons and stents, etc.), especially the application of a series of products with small diameters and long balloons dedicated to lower extremity arteries, the long-segment occlusion lesions and infra-knee arteries significantly improved clinical efficacy. For diabetic inferior knee arterial disease, the technical success rate of PTA alone is 86%, the 1-year patency rate is 53–56%, and the limb salvage rate is 81–85%. The 1-year patency rate is 54%, and the limb salvage rate is 97.1%, but there is a risk of contrast-related nephropathy, especially in patients with potential or renal insufficiency, the incidence is higher and the prognosis is poor. Therefore, for patients with ischemic ulcers, when clinically considering the use of percutaneous intravascular interventional therapy, adequate hydration should be performed and the changes in renal function of the patients should be closely monitored.

If autologous vascular bypass is performed, a good saphenous vein is also required. By-pass surgery using autologous blood vessels, the 5-year patency rate was 63%, and the salvage rate was 78%. For the treatment of sub-knee occlusion with saphenous vein bypass, the patency rates at 1 and 3 years were 63 and 50%, and the salvage rates were 85 and 79%. When the foot disease further develops and leads to irreversible ischemic necrosis of the limb, or necrosis of the affected limb with serious infection that cannot be controlled, directly threatens the patient's life, or the long-term spasm of the distal small artery due to severe peripheral neuritis causes the limb to become distant. For patients with end-stage ischemic necrosis, amputation is not only a treatment method, but more importantly, it can save the patient's life. For diabetic foot amputation, the amputation plane should be reduced as much as possible on the premise of ensuring the amputation effect, and arteriography should be performed before the amputation to determine the amputation plane.

4.4 Multidisciplinary collaborative therapy

The systematic review shows that multidisciplinary team collaboration therapy can focus on the advantages of various professions, which has a positive impact on shortening wound healing time, reducing amputation rate and reducing the severity of amputation [23]. The treatment of diabetic foot requires clinical multi-disciplinary collaboration. The diabetic specialist first evaluates the patient's systemic condition to minimize the occurrence of cardiovascular complications; at the same time evaluates vascular conditions and creates percutaneous vascular intraluminal intervention treatment or surgical treatment conditions, discuss operative methods with vascular surgery and endovascular interventional physicians, orthopedic physicians, make rescue plans for intraoperative and postoperative cardiovascular events, and follow-up and drug adjustment after successful surgery. Only in this way can the blood circulation reconstruction of diabetic foot patients be improved to the greatest extent, and amputation and death rates can be reduced. Early and timely multi-disciplinary collaborative treatment is also recommended by the domestic 2017 version of the guidelines.

A multi-disciplinary team of diabetic foot medical care professionals can effectively reduce the rate of diabetic amputation and medical expenses, and improve the quality of life of patients. In the recently reported 240,000 rural areas of England, after the establishment of a multidisciplinary team of diabetic foot led by vascular surgery experts, the amputation rate of diabetic lower limbs decreased from 412 per 100,000 to 15–44 per 100,000 [24]. The changes in medical services are reflected in: increasing the community's awareness and clinical path to this multidisciplinary collaborative podiatry team service, as far as possible, patients are admitted to specialty wards, a rapid referral channel, an operation room in the outpatient department for debridement, small amputation; a podiatrist, orthopedics and vascular surgery joint outpatient clinic; the hospital's senior podiatrist and community podiatrist have a network of links to pay attention to diabetic patients. For patients who need to strengthen outpatient follow-up, implement weekly or 2 weeks, a joint outpatient clinic; hospital specialists and nurses follow up the patients closely to achieve clinical follow-up at the patients' homes. The French medical management department requires that patients with diabetic foot must be referred to a hospital with a diabetic foot care team within 48 hours.

4.5 Stem cell transplantation for diabetic foot disease

Despite the rapid development of endovascular interventional techniques and surgical techniques, there are still some patients with ischemic foot disease can't receive interventional or surgical treatment. This part of patients is called "no Treatment Options for Patients. Recent clinical trials on autologous stem cell transplantation for lower limb ischemia have achieved satisfactory results. Tateishi-Yuyama et al. [25]. reported for the first time that bone marrow stem cell transplantation was used to treat patients with peripheral vascular disease, local autologous bone marrow mesenchymal stem cells were sprayed locally on chronic ulcers with a duration of more than 1 year. The wounds began to close after 2–4 weeks, and the wound healing rate was proportional to the number of stem cells; a 3-year follow-up of patients with autologous bone marrow mononuclear stem cell transplantation for the treatment of arterial ischemic diseases of the lower extremities showed that this treatment can improve the ischemia of the lower extremities for a long time and prolong the survival time of the affected limbs. Lu et al. also confirmed that bone marrow mononuclear stem cells and bone marrow mesenchymal stem cells can promote ulcer healing, prolong the claudication distance, increase ankle brachial index and percutaneous oxygen partial pressure in patients with diabetic foot, however, the effect of latter is better than the former. In addition, the combined application of stem cell transplantation and interventional therapy can make up for their respective shortcomings, and benefit more than a single method. Therefore, for patients with "no treatment options", consider referral to a qualified medical unit for autologous stem cell transplantation treatment. Although this treatment method is still under exploration and research, it is still its hope for future treatment.

5. Follow-up of diabetic foot

Peripheral neuropathy, lower extremity arterial disease (LEAD), and foot deformities are the main reasons for the increased risk of DFU. Age, gender, education, economic conditions, lifestyle habits and other complications or complications of diabetes are also important factors. Fully understanding these factors is very important for the risk assessment of diabetic foot and taking corresponding preventive measures.

The patient's quality of life is low, mental and psychological pressure is high, and the medical cost burden is heavy. Therefore, early evaluation to prevent foot ulcers and timely cure of ulcers to prevent recurrence, thereby avoiding amputations or large amputations above the ankle joint, is the focus of DF tertiary prevention.

It is generally believed that the preventive measures against DF should be divided into three levels. Primary prevention is to identify and avoid the risk factors that lead to DF as early as possible to prevent its occurrence; secondary prevention is to identify DF as early as possible and prevent its progress; tertiary prevention is to ensure appropriate treatment of DF.

5.1 Periodic inspections for DF high-risk factors

The main risk factors for DF include diabetic peripheral neuropathy, foot deformity, peripheral vascular disease, foot ulcer history, foot amputation or leg amputation history. According to the recommendations of the International Diabetes Foot Working Group (IWGDF), for patients with diabetes without high-risk factors, a foot examination should be performed by a specialist at least once a year. For patients with high-risk factors, more frequent inspections should be conducted according to the category of high-risk factors, in order to detect these high-risk factors and their progress as soon as possible, and provide patients with appropriate measures to prevent foot ulcers [26].

5.2 Health education

Systematic diabetic foot related knowledge education can reduce the incidence of DFU, reduce the recurrence rate of DFU and improve the survival rate of foot-less ulcer events, reduce the amputation rate of DFU, reduce medical expenses and improve the quality of life of patients [27, 28]. Diabetic foot specialist medical staff educates patients and their families on foot protection knowledge and nursing, and helps them transform into effective actions [29]. Although there are few clinical studies that specifically assess whether health education can prevent DFU, and the level of evidence is low [30], these health education measures can enable patients to detect early lesions of DFU, strengthen self-behavior management, and keep feet clean which are important means to prevent ulcer occurrence and recurrence [31].

Predictors of DF amputation or re-amputation include adult males, long-term diabetes, wound infections, diabetic neuropathy, and smoking history [32]. DF occurs mostly in manual workers, patients are generally less educated, lack knowledge of diabetes prevention, lack of awareness of the severity of its complications, and pay insufficient attention to early blood glucose control and DF prevention. Therefore, we must pay attention to the health education of diabetic patients, so that they have a full understanding of the development and outcome of the disease, so as to actively cooperate with prevention, such as actively quitting smoking, controlling blood sugar, doing daily foot inspections, and doing foot protection., Foot care, pay attention to toenail trimming and comfortable footwear, etc., in order to detect and avoid the risk factors of DF as early as possible, to prevent the formation of ulcers, infections and further development.

5.3 Local load reduction measures

Qualified DF protective shoes can significantly reduce the incidence of foot ulcers. The custom-made DF protective shoes generally have the following functions: protect the sense of loss from external damage; adapt to the deformity of the foot to reduce pain and prevent the increase of the deformity of the foot; reduce excessive local pressure, so that the pressure is evenly distributed; reduce shear force in vertical and horizontal direction [33]. Multiple studies have shown that wearing foot protection shoes can effectively reduce plantar pressure by about 30%. Compared with wearing ordinary shoes, the risk of foot ulcer recurrence in DF patients is reduced by 46.1–70.2%. For patients with high-risk feet with hammer-toe diabetes who are not ideal for the use of conservative measures such as protective shoes, distal flexor tendon amputation can prevent the formation of tip toe ulcers, and its cost performance and risk-benefit ratio are encouraging [34].

For diabetic patients with risk factors for podiatry, early completion of diabetes peripheral neuropathy (DPN), vascular disease and podiatry screening, early detection and management of these high-risk patients are needed. Non-diabetic foot medical staff should refer to the diabetic foot specialist or consult with the specialist in a timely manner for patients with the following conditions: sharp changes in skin color, increased local pain and inflammation such as redness, new ulcers, original There are superficial ulcers that deteriorate and involve soft tissue and/or bone tissue, disseminated cellulitis, signs of systemic infection, osteomyelitis, etc. Timely referral or consultation can help reduce the amputation rate and reduce medical costs, and timely intervention of the surgeon can help reduce the diabetic amputation rate and amputation plane.

Therefore, it is currently emphasized that for patients with diabetes, screening of lower extremity arterial diseases should be strengthened to achieve early diagnosis and early treatment. For patients with moderate to severe lower extremity arterial disease and complete foot skin, it is recommended to guide the patient to exercise rehabilitation exercise for at least 3–6 months, but for patients with foot skin ulcers, it is recommended to brake and avoid exercise rehabilitation At the same time, it is recommended to use low-dose aspirin, statin lipid-lowering drugs, angiotensin-converting enzyme inhibitors, vasodilator drugs and anticoagulant drugs, which can reduce the occurrence of ulcers and improve patients' lower limb motor function.

Acknowledgements

This work was financially supported by "Graduate education innovation program project of Guangdong province" (No. 2020XLLT10) and "Twenty-one teaching reform projects of Jinan University" (No. JG2019044). The funding body supported the team to design the study and collection, analysis, and interpretation of data and write the manuscript.

Conflict of interest

The authors declare no conflict of interest.

Author details

Fanna Liu* and Lianghong Yin
Nephrology Department, The First Affiliated Hospital of Jinan University, Guangzhou, China

*Address all correspondence to: tliufana@jnu.edu.cn

References

[1] Lu B, Hu J, Wen J, et al. Determination of peripheral neuropathy prevalence and associated factors in Chinese subjects with diabetes and pre-diabetes -ShangHai diabetic neuRopathy epidemiology and molecular genetics study (SH-DREAMS). PLoS One. 2013;**8**(4):e61053. DOI: 10.1371/journal.pone.0061053

[2] Bakker K, Apelqvist J, Lipsky BA, et al. The 2015 IWGDF guidance documents on prevention and management of foot problems in diabetes: Development of an evidence-based global consensus. Diabetes/Metabolism Research and Reviews. 2016;**32**(Suppl 1):S2-S6

[3] Skrepnek GH, Mills JL Sr, Lavery LA, et al. Health care service and outcomes among an estimated 6.7 million ambulatory care diabetic foot cases in the U. S. Diabetes Care. 2017;**40**(7):936-942. DOI: 10.2337/dc16-2189

[4] Margolis DJ, Malay DS, Hoffstad OJ, et al. Incidence of Diabetic Foot Ulcer and Lower Extremity Amputation among Medicare Beneficiaries, 2006 to 2008. Rockville (MD): Agency for Healthcare Research and Quality (US); 2011

[5] International Diabetes Federation. IDF Diabetes Atlas, 8th.Brussels: 2017[EB/OL]. Available from: http://www.diabetesatlas.org [Accessed: 02 January 2019]

[6] Raghav A, Khan ZA, Labala RK, et al. Financial burden of diabetic foot ulcers to world: A progressive topic to discuss always. Therapeutic Advances in Endocrinology and Metabolism. 2018;**9**(1):29-31. DOI: 10.1177/2042018817744513

[7] Driver VR, Fabbi M, Lavery LA, et al. The costs of diabetic foot: The economic case for the limb salvage team. Journal of Vascular Surgery. 2010;**52**(3 Suppl):S17-S22. DOI: 10.1016/j.jvs.2010.06.003

[8] Wagner FW Jr. The diabetic foot. Orthopedics. 1987;**10**:163-172

[9] Lavery LA, Armstrong DG, Harkless LB. Classification of diabetic foot wounds. The Journal of Foot and Ankle Surgery. 1996;**35**:528-613

[10] Bonnet C, Carello C, Turvey MT. Diabetes and postural stability: Review and hypAssociation AD. Standards of medical care in diabetes-2006. Diabetes Care. 2006;**30**(Suppl 1):S4-S42

[11] Khairoun M, van den Heuvel M, van den Berg BM, et al. Early systemic microvascular damage in pigs with atherogenic diabetes mellitus coincides with renal angiopoietin dysbalance. PLoS One. 2015;**10**(4):e0121555

[12] Association AD. Standards of medical care in diabetes-2006. Diabetes Care. 2006;**30**(Suppl 1):S4-S42

[13] Hasan R, Firwana B, Elraiyah T, et al. A systematic review and meta analysis of glycemic control for the prevention of diabetic foot syndrome. Journal of Vascular Surgery. 2016;**63**(s2):22-28

[14] Zhang SS, Tang ZY, Fang P, et al. Nutritional status deteriorates as the severity of diabetic foot ulcers increases and independently associates with prognosis. Experimental and Therapeutic Medicine. 2013;**5**(1):215-222

[15] Acar E, Kaclra BK. Predictors of lower extremity amputation and reamputation in the diabetic foot. The Journal of Foot and Ankle Surgery. 2017;**56**:1218-1222

[16] Zhao Z, Ji L, Zheng L, et al. Effectiveness of clinical alternatives to nerve conduction studies for screening for diabetic distal symmetrical polyneuropathy: A multi-center study. Diabetes Research and Clinical Practice. 2016;**115**:150-156. DOI: 10.1016/j.diabres.2016.01

[17] Ndosi M, Wright-Hughes A, Brown S, et al. Prognosis of the infected diabetic foot ulcer: A 12-month prospective observational study. Diabetic Medicine. 2018;**35**(1):78-88

[18] Serra R, Grande R, Butrico L, et al. Chronic wound infections: The role of Pseudomonas aeruginosa and Staphylococcus aureus. Expert Review of Anti-Infective Therapy. 2015;**13**(5):605-613. DOI: 10.1586/14787210.2015.1023291

[19] Lipsky BA, Berendt AR, Cornia PB, et al. 2012 infectious diseases society of America clinical practice guideline for the diagnosis and treatment of diabetic foot infections. Journal of the American Podiatric Medical Association. 2013;**103**(1):2-7

[20] Qi M, Zhou Q, Zeng W, et al. Growth factors in the pathogenesis of diabetic foot ulcers. Frontiers in Bioscience. 2018;**23**:310-317

[21] Barrientos S, Brem H, Stojadinovic O, et al. Clinical application of growth factors and cytokines in wound healing. Wound Repair and Regeneration. 2014;**22**(5):569-578. DOI: 10.1111/wrr.12205

[22] Sridharan K, Sivaramakrishnan G. Growth factors for diabetic foot ulcers: Mixed treatment comparison analysis of randomized clinical trials. British Journal of Clinical Pharmacology. 2018;**84**(3):434-444. DOI: 10.1111/bcp.13470

[23] Buggy A, Moore Z. The impact of the multidisciplinary team in the management of individuals with diabetic foot ulcers: A systematic review. Journal of Wound Care. 2017;**26**(6):324-339

[24] Williams DT, Powell-Chandler A, Qureshi Q, et al. Improved limb salvage for patients with vascular disease and tissue loss associated with new model of provision targeted at the diabetic foot. Diabetes Research and Clinical Practice. 2018;**135**:50-57. DOI: 10.1016/j.diabres.2017.10.015

[25] Tateishi-Yuyama E, Matsubara H, Murohara T, et al. Therapeutic angiogenesis for patients with limb ischaemia by autologous transplantation of bone-marrow cells: A pilot study and a randomised controlled trial. Lancet. 2002;**360**(9331):427-435. DOI: 10.1016/S0140-6736(02)09670-8

[26] Bus SA, van Netten JJ, Lavery LA, et al. IWGDF guidance on the prevention of foot ulcers in at-risk patients with diabetes. Diabetes/Metabolism Research and Reviews. 2016;**32**(S1):16-24

[27] Ren M, Yang C, Lin DZ, et al. Effect of intensive nursing education on the prevention of diabetic foot ulceration among patients with high-risk diabetic foot: A follow-up analysis. Diabetes Technology & Therapeutics. 2014;**16**(9):576-581. DOI: 10.1089/dia.2014.0004

[28] Dorresteijn JA, Kriegsman DM, Assendelft WJ, et al. Patient education for preventing diabetic foot ulceration. Cochrane Database of Systematic Reviews. 2014;**12**:CD001488. DOI: 10.1002/14651858.CD001488

[29] Rerkasem K, Kosachunhanun N, Tongprasert S, Guntawongwan K. A multidisciplinary diabetic foot protocol at Chiang Mai University Hospital: Cost and quality of life.

The International Journal of Lower Extremity Wounds. 2009;**8**(3):153-156. DOI: 10.1177/1534734609344143

[30] Dargis V, Pantelejeva O, Jonushaite A, et al. Benefits of amultidisciplinary approach in the management of recurrent diabetic foot ulceration in Lithuania: A prospective study. Diabetes Care. 1999;**22**(9):1428-1431

[31] Vedhara K, Beattie A, Metcalfe C, et al. Development and preliminary evaluation of a psychosocial intervention for modifying psychosocial risk factors associated with foot reulceration in diabetes. Behaviour Research and Therapy. 2012;**50**(5):323-332. DOI: 10.1016/j.brat.2012.02.013

[32] Acar E, Kaclra BK. Predictors of lower extremity amputation and reamputation in the diabetic foot. The Journal of Foot and Ankle Surgery. 2017;**56**:1218-1222

[33] Ulbrecht JS, Hurley T, Mauger DT, et al. Prevention of recurrent foot ulcers with plantar pressure-based in-shoe orthoses: The careful prevention multicenter randomized controlled trial. Diabetes Care. 2014;**37**(7):1982-1989

[34] Tamir E, Vigler M, Avisar E, et al. Percutaneous tenotomy for the treatment of diabetic toe ulcers. Foot & Ankle International. 2014;**35**(1):38-43

Chapter 11

Neurocognitive Dysfunction and Diabetic Foot

Caroline A. Fisher

Abstract

Diabetic foot ulcers are one of the most serious complications associated with diabetes. People with diabetes experience an accelerated rate of age-related cognitive decline, and comorbid complications increase the likelihood of neurocognitive attenuation. The current body of research into neurocognitive functioning in individuals with diabetic foot ulcers is small, but suggests significantly increased rates of neurocognitive dysfunction, and that up to one quarter of this cohort have cognitive functioning consistent with dementia samples. This has implications for utilising disease self-management as the primary treatment model. Neurocognitive deficits mean that understanding, retaining, and adhering to management recommendations are likely to be difficult in this group. Further research is needed in this area to determine the specific neurocognitive profile associated with diabetic foot, including which cognitive domains are the most impacted. The provision of a framework for tailoring management strategies to assist this group with more efficacious disease management is also required.

Keywords: cognition, diabetic, diabetic foot, neurocognitive functioning, neuropsychology, self-management, ulcers

1. Introduction

Diabetes mellitus is a disorder of insulin deficiency and is categorised into two types. The primary mechanism of disease in Type 1 is the loss of pancreatic islet β-cells [1], resulting in an inability to produce insulin. The typical trio of onset of symptoms for Type 1 are excess thirst, increased appetite, and excess urine production, as well as overt hyperglycaemia [2]. The definitive cause of Type 1 diabetes is not known. However, it is believed that it is likely to be related to an immune or auto-immune system disorder in 70–90% of those affected (Type 1A), with remainder of cases considered idiopathic (Type 1B) [2]. Type 1 is most commonly diagnosed in childhood, although onset can occur at any age [2]. Type 1 is estimated to account for 5–15% of all cases of diabetes [1]. There is no cure for the condition and individuals with this disorder require the injection of insulin to survive [3].

Type 2 diabetes is generally triggered by a number of lifestyle factors including being overweight or obese, having a sedentary lifestyle and consuming a diet containing high amounts of processed and red meat, refined grains and drinks that are high in sugar [4]. It shares many of the symptoms of type 1, and also involves progressive pancreatic β-cell failure. The initial phases are characterised by changes in the bodies' response to insulin and can later progress to insufficient insulin being produced [3]. However, it has been indicated that the mechanisms that trigger β-cell death via cytokine and nutrient changes in Type 2 are different from those that occur in Type 1 [5]. In contrast to Type 1, Type 2 diabetes can be controlled by dietary changes and oral medication, but can require the need for the injection of exogenous insulin with progression and worsening of the disease [3].

Type 1 diabetes is the most common type in children, with Type 2 very rare in those under 30 years of age [3]. The onset of Type 2 diabetes most commonly occurs in adulthood and is the most prevalent type of diabetes. Rates of both types appear to be growing with a global rise in all forms of diabetes noted over the last 40 years with the greatest magnitude of increase thought to be driven by adult Type 2 cases [6, 7]. Thus, the health burden of diabetes is becoming more pronounced, increasing the strain on health systems and resulting in an upturn in diabetes related disease burden across the world.

1.1 Diabetes complications: foot ulcers

Diabetic foot ulcers are one of the most serious complications of the disease as they can lead to amputation [8], significantly increasing disease burden [9]. They are more common in people with peripheral arterial disease, and are generally caused by repeated pressure on an area that has high rates of vertical or sheer stress in people who suffer from peripheral neuropathy [10]. Healing of foot wounds can be slow, particularly if management guidelines are not followed, with 23% of wounds still present, after 12 months [11]. Foot ulcers can occur in people with both Type 1 and Type 2 diabetes. A recent systematic review indicated that the global rate of foot ulcers in people with diabetes is 6.3% [12]. Although variance in regional prevalence rates was found, with North America and Africa having the highest rates and Europe and Oceania the lowest [12]. Individuals who develop diabetic foot ulcers tend to have a longer duration of diabetic exposure, and higher rates of hypertension, diabetic retinopathy and smoking, but lower body mass indexes [12]. Diabetic foot ulcers occur prior to lower extremity amputations in around 84% of cases, and are associated with an increased risk of death by almost two and a half times, compared to people with diabetes without ulcers [13–15]. Research utilising a large Australian sample recently indicated a five-year mortality rate of 24.6% and a 10 year mortality rate of 45.4% in individuals treated at a multi-disciplinary foot clinic for diabetic foot ulcers [16]. Foot ulcers are also consistently shown to be associated with a significant decrease in quality of life, impacting on many lifestyle areas including social functioning, employment, financial security, interpersonal relationships, psychological and physical health [17, 18].

1.2 Diabetes complications: neurological abnormalities

Despite being anatomically located at opposite ends of the body, foot ulcers and changes in brain functioning have a number of similar predisposing factors in individuals with diabetes. Co-occurring hypertension, diabetic retinopathy and current smoking are correlated with higher rates of neurological abnormalities observed through brain imaging in people with diabetes [19–21]. A systematic review of the diabetes brain imaging literature by van Harten et al. in 2006 included 55 studies the majority with predominantly middle age to early elderly cohort [22]. The review indicated that lacunar infarcts and cerebral atrophy are associated with diabetes, but that an association with white-matter lesions was unclear, due to the poor quality of the available studies in detecting subtle abnormalities of this kind. A narrative review from 2014 suggested that Type 1 diabetes was associated with small alterations in brain volume in specific areas, including frontal, temporal and posterior cortical areas, as well as subcortical grey matter [23]. These changes appear to occur early, with volumetric changes in Type 1 diabetes detectable, relative to controls, in childhood. In Type 2 diabetes volumetric loss is also observed but tends to be most commonly found in cortical and subcortical areas surrounding the ventricles [23]. While smaller hippocampal volumes have been found, this has generally been commensurate with the magnitude of total volume loss, and thus specific atrophy of hippocampal areas (which have relevance to memory) in diabetes is not definitive.

A recent a systematic review of dynamic brain imaging investigated task and resting-state fMRI functional magnetic resonance imaging (fMRI) in diabetes. It concluded that reductions in the default mode network (DMN) connectivity are associated with diabetes [24]. The DMN is the brain network that is engaged when individuals are not actively participating in task-based pursuits (i.e. 'at rest'). Findings of abnormal network activity during task based studies were reported to be less consistent, with some studies reporting reduced brain activation in brain areas related to the task, and others over activation [24]. Neurological changes in diabetes have relevance to neurocognitive functioning and this association will be explored further in Section 2.2.

1.3 Diabetes self-management

The impact of diabetes on health, wellbeing and functioning can be seen, from head to toe, with the effect of non-optimal management of the disease having significant implications for quality of life and morbidity. The importance of diabetes self-management has been promoted within the field as a means to assist individuals with diabetes to manage their condition effectively and minimise complications [25–28]. Best practice self-management support has been identified as including; education about diabetes and treatment options; managing nutrition and exercise as part of on-going lifestyle changes; utilising prescribed medications safety to maximise their therapeutic efficacy; self-monitoring of factors such as blood glucose levels and using effective decision making to interpret the results; employing strategies to manage complications, detecting these when they do arise and treating them early and appropriately; identifying and managing psychosocial issues; and developing strategies to promote health and behaviour change that will be effective for the individual [25]. Many of these self-management strategies require a range of higher level cognitive skills to be implemented and maintained consistently. However, neurocognitive attention is associated with the disease, and neurocognitive difficulties may impact on the capacity of individuals with diabetes to effectively implement disease self-management strategies.

2. Neurocognitive functioning in diabetes

Neurocognitive abilities are localised in the brain and encompass a broad range of thinking skills including attention, concentration, processing speed, new learning and memory, language, planning, organisation, problem solving and visual-perceptual and spatial abilities. In addition to looking at skills in specific neurocognitive domains, overall measures of ability, such as intellectual assessment (IQ) can also be conducted to provide information about general cognitive functioning. Neurocognitive skills impact on daily living and deficits can effect an individual's functional and vocational capacity. Neurocognitive deficits are defining features of a number of neurological cognitions, including dementia and traumatic brain injuries, and the assessment and management of these difficulties falls within the specialty of clinical neuropsychology.

2.1 Theory of neurocognitive functioning across the lifespan in diabetes and complications

There is a relatively large body of literature that has investigated the impact of diabetes on neurocognitive functioning. In 2008, Biessels and colleagues hypothesised a framework for conceptualising the impact of diabetes on neurocognition, across the lifespan [3]. Following a thorough review of the literature available at the time, they proposed two age-related time point vulnerabilities for diabetes to detrimentally impact on neurocognitive functioning, with additional further increased risk observed in individuals with high levels of co-morbid diabetes related complications. Biessels et al. proposed that the first time period for cognitive attenuation vulnerability was during the period of neuronal maturation and brain development in childhood [3]. They suggested that those children who developed Type 1 diabetes at a younger age (i.e. between 5 and 7 years) were at higher risk of showing attenuated cognitive development, compared those who developed Type 1 later in childhood. The second age-related period of increased vulnerability to cognitive attenuation was proposed to occur at the time point were normal age-related cognitive decline begins across several cognitive domains, in middle age. Biessels et al. suggested that individuals with diabetes in middle and older age (predominantly a Type 2 cohort) are likely to show an accelerated rate of cognitive decline, relative to their age matched peers [3]. Diabetes related co-morbidities were proposed as a third variable that increased the risk of cognitive attenuation in diabetes cohorts. The primary conditions posited in this area were microvascular disease, severe hypoglycemic episodes, and hypertension [3].

The hypothesis outlined by Biessels et al. [3], continues to hold merit since it was first proposed, with subsequent findings that have been published in the last 10 years largely supporting this framework. Longitudinal data from Type 1 diabetes research (following individuals with childhood diagnoses through to youth, at 12 years follow-up) has indicated that early onset is associated with poorer sustained attention, divided attention, new learning, and mental efficiency [29]. Longitudinal data from ageing studies has indicated that in middle aged cohorts accelerated cognitive decline is observed in those who had Type 2 diabetes at study baseline, relative to non-diabetes age-matched peers [30]. Additionally, incident diabetes (those who go on to develop diabetes but have not been diagnosed at baseline) showed subtle early decline in information processing speed, which became more pronounced following diagnosis and with increasing duration of illness [30]. The Biessels et al. proposal [3] that higher rates of diabetes complications increases the risk of cognitive decline has also been supported, with several studies showing greater rates of neurocognitive attenuation in people with diabetes who also have hypertension, neuropathy, retinopathy [30–32].

Recent research has also indicated a link between diabetes, neurocognitive decline and dementia, and that the link may be stronger in women [23, 33–35]. The primary dementia syndromes associated with diabetes are Alzheimer's disease and vascular dementia. It has been suggested that the neuropathogenesis in diabetes and Alzheimer's disease may be related, and that the increased burden of small-vessel disease in diabetes can contribute to the development of a vascular based dementia [23, 33]. Dementia, as defined under the Major Neurocognitive Disorder framework within Diagnostic and Statistical Manual of Mental Disorders, is primarily a disorder of neurocognitive dysfunction [36]. As such, it is not surprising that capacity for disease self-management in people with diabetes and co-occurring dementia is diminished [33]. It has been posited that there is a bidirectional impact, whereby poor self-management, due to cognitive impairment from dementia, leads to poorer diabetes control, increasing the likelihood of further cognitive impairment [33].

As such, further investigation is needed into how to specifically target education and management strategies in this group, as they may not be able to utilise these in the same way as those with stronger neurocognitive functioning.

2.2 Neurocognitive profile in diabetes

Not all studies separate Type 1 and Type 2 diabetes cases when investigating neurocognitive functioning in adults. Where the types have been looked at individually, or in studies where the research has demarked the groups discretely, there are both similarities and differences in the profile of cognitive attenuation [37]. A systematic review of the Type 1 literature was conducted in 2005 and included 33 studies [38]. This review indicated that Type 1 diabetes is associated with attenuation in functioning on overall intelligence measures, as well as attention, psychomotor processing speed, cognitive flexibility and visual-perceptual and spatial functioning at the domain level [37, 38]. Notably however, the mean age of participants in studies included in this review most commonly fell in the 30s, with the oldest mean age of 47.6 years. Thus, the review data was mainly comprised of younger adult cohorts, and relatively little is known about the Type 1 neurocognitive profile in middle aged and older adults.

Type 2 diabetes cohorts show some similarities in their neurocognitive profile to Type 1. They exhibit attenuation in their processing speed, attention and executive functioning, but tend show a greater magnitude of decrement in memory functioning compared to Type 1 [30, 37, 39]. There is presently no seminal, overarching systematic review and meta-analysis that has attempted to synthesise the evidence base regarding cognitive functioning in adults with Type 2 diabetes, relative to controls, across all major neurocognitive domains. The most comprehensive attempt to integrate the literature was a meta-analysis published by Palta and colleagues in in 2014. This meta-analysis looked at neurocognitive functioning in six areas, across 24 studies with a total of 3351 patients with diabetes [40]. The included studies were predominantly from western countries, and there was a relatively large age range between the studies with means in the late 50s to early 80s. The results indicated that at a domain level, the largest effect size for diabetes status was seen in the areas of motor function ($d = -0.36$), executive function ($d = -0.33$) and processing speed ($d = -0.33$), followed by verbal memory ($d = -0.28$), visual memory ($d = 0.26$) and attention/concentration ($d = -0.19$). Specific neurocognitive tests were also identified that were most likely to demonstrate diabetes related cognitive attenuation. These included the dominant hand condition on the Grooved Pegboard, immediate recall on the Rey Auditory Verbal Learning Task, trails A and B from The Trail Making Test, delayed recall from the Rey-Osterreith Complex Figure task, and part 1 of the Stroop task. The research team did note, however that they were unable to stratify the results according to age, could not make any comments in regard to gender, and also noted that the results may not be representative across different ethnicity groups.

Task based fMRI studies have indicated that alterations in activation networks may be correlated with performance levels on neuropsychological assessment [24]. There is some evidence that poorer memory performances are seen in individuals with diabetes who have reduced activation in the default mode network [41]. Reduced speed on a complex trail making activity requiring set-shifting (trails B) and complex figure delayed recall has been associated with neural abnormalities in the cuneus and lingual gyrus, areas associated with inhibitory control and visual memory [42]. Thus, there is some evidence linking functional brain activation changes and poorer neuropsychological functioning in this population.

3. Neurocognitive functioning in individuals with diabetic foot ulcers

Relative to the general diabetes literature, fewer research studies have been conducted that have investigated neurocognitive functioning specifically in people with diabetes and foot ulcers [43–46]. The research that is available appears to indicate attenuated functioning, at a group level, and significant impairments in a proportion of patients. This section of the chapter reviews what is known about neurocognitive functioning in people with diabetic foot ulcers and provides suggestions for future research.

3.1 Cognitive screening and diabetic foot

Cognitive screening measures are short, easy to administer assessments that provide an overall measure of basic cognitive functioning. They generally require limited or short-duration training to administer and are utilised by a wide range of clinical disciplines. One of the most commonly administered cognitive screening measures is the Mini Mental State Examination (MMSE) [47]. A study by Marseglia et al. [43] utilised the MMSE to investigate cognitive functioning in a moderately sized cohort (n = 153) of individuals with diabetic foot complications. The sample was predominantly male (75.8%). The mean age of the cohort was 65 years (SD 10.5) and the authors further sub-grouped this cohort into patients aged under 65 years (n = 73) and those aged over 65 years (n = 80). HbA1c levels were reported at a mean of 7.7 (SD 1.4). The medium length of diabetes duration was 20 years, and a high proportion (70.6%) had undergone amputation.

In the Marseglia, et al. study [43] the mean MMSE score was found to be 24.6 (SD = 3.6), with a range of 11–30. The authors used the cut-off score derived by Kivipelto et al. [48], with scores $\leq$24 defined as being indicative of general cognitive function impairment. Using this criterion, 39% of the total sample demonstrated cognitive impairment. The was a significant difference by age stratification with 25% of the patients below 65 years showing impairment, compared to 53% of those above 65 years. Logistic regression indicated that foot amputation was associated with lower MMSE scores. No information was provided about which items/domains within the MMSE assessment were more commonly impaired. However, a small range of additional cognitive assessment measures were also employed in this study, and these will be reported, by domain, in Section 3.2.

A recently published study by Corbett and colleagues investigated neurocognitive functioning in individuals with diabetic foot ulcers using a newer, and increasingly widely used, cognitive screening measure, the Montreal Cognitive Assessment (MoCA) [45]. The like the MMSE, the MoCA is a quick (5–10 min) assessment tool that provides an overview of cognitive functioning, and is designed to detect cognitive decline. The MoCA provides better coverage of executive functioning, and higher-level language and visuospatial processing, relative to the MMSE, and produces less of a ceiling effect (i.e. is harder overall) [49]. The study by Corbett et al. [45] reported on MoCA and Patient Interpretation of Neuropathy (PIN) data in 30 patients with diabetic foot ulcers admitted to a specialist hospital unit for inpatient management of their foot wounds. The mean age of the study cohort was later middle age (m = 58.37 years, 10.64 SD), and the sample predominantly male (83%). Most of the cohort had type 2 diabetes (93%) of between 1 and 38 years duration (mode 10 years). The mean HBA1C level was 9.27 (SD 2.45), and there were high rates of macrovascular disease (60%) and hypertension (47%), moderate rates of nephropathy (27%) and retinopathy (23%). Thus, the cohort was younger than in the Marseglia et al. [43] study, but with poorer diabetes control, based on HbA1c results.

The education corrected total mean MoCA score in the Corbett et al. [45], study was 22.37 (SD 3.65), and range 12 to 27, with no patients achieving a full score of 30/30. Recommended MoCA cut-off scores to demark mild cognitive impairment vary from study to study [50–53]. Thus, the authors provided the percentages of participants below the full range of suggested cut-of values. A total of 87% of the cohort fell below the stringent cut-off criteria of <27, a further 77% below <26 and 43% below <23. Further, 27% of the sample had a total MoCA score of <20. This indicates that more than one quarter of diabetic foot ulcer patients in this study had a MoCA score consistent with diagnosed dementia cohorts [52, 53]. When separated into individual cognitive areas, patients most commonly made errors on items assessing short-term recall (90%), executive functioning (87%) and language (77%), while in contrast items assessing orientation showed the highest degree of accuracy (90% scoring full marks).

The results of this study also reported on patients' interpretations of their neuropathy on the PIN. Correlation analysis indicated that patients with higher MoCA scores provided more accurate responses on the Acute Foot Ulcer Onset PIN subscale. This subscale measures knowledge about how foot ulcers can develop. Thus, individuals with diabetic foot ulcers and lower cognitive functioning may have reduced understanding of how foot wounds occur.

The Australian MoCA results from the Corbett et al. [45] study can be further compared with existing studies that have used the MoCA for cognitive screening assessment in other diabetes cohorts [31, 54, 55], see **Table 1**. Participants in one of the comparison studies were Japanese inpatients receiving training on diabetes management [31], in another they were Canadian patients at diabetes education clinics [55], and in the third it is not reported where the Turkish subject group were recruited from [54]. In each comparison study foot ulcer status was not commented on, but prevalence could be expected to parallel that of global estimates of foot ulcers in people with diabetes at around 6%, with a range between 2 and 14% consistent with prevalence rates found in each of the study countries [12].

The results displayed in **Table 1** suggest that cognitive attenuation in diabetic foot ulcer individuals exceeds expectation, based on their diabetes status and age. The mean MoCA scores obtained by individuals with diabetic foot ulcers in the Corbett et al. [45] study were higher than those reported by Ozcan et al. [54] However, the mean age of the Ozcan et al. [50] study group was 13 years older. The Corbett et al. [45] MoCA results were similar to the Mori et al. [31] results—a group that had comparable HbA1c scores but a higher mean age, by 9 years. Compared to the cohort with the closest age match, Alagiakrishnan et al. [55] the Corbett et al. [43] MoCA results were notably lower.

Lead author, study year	Ozcan, 2014	Mori, 2015	Alagiakrishnan, 2013	Corbett, 2019
Mean age (SD)	71.27 (8.57)	67.3 (9.9)	59.9 (7.1)	58.37 (10.64)
Sample size	15	29	30	30
Mean HbA1c (SD)	N/A	9.6 (1.8)	N/A	9.27 (2.45)
Foot ulcer status	N/A	N/A	N/A	100%
MoCA mean (SD)	15.53 (6.18)	22.87 (3.80)*	26.45 (2.72)*	22.37 (3.65)

**Total cohort Mean and SD calculated from pooled MCI present and MCI absent groups.*

Table 1.
Comparison of MoCA Cognitive Screening scores in Older Diabetes Cohorts.

3.2 Neuropsychological assessment and diabetic foot

Screening measures such as the MoCA and similar measures like the MMSE are useful as quick and easy to administer assessments, providing an overview of cognitive functioning [56]. They are designed to identify patients who may be experiencing cognitive decline but are limited in their capacity to pin-point specific cognitive deficits and the magnitude of neurocognitive attenuation, relative to estimated premorbid cognitive functioning. Neuropsychological assessments are the gold standard for eliciting this type of in-depth information on neurocognitive functioning, and ideally, where access is available, individuals with reduced scoring on cognitive screening measures should be referred for neuropsychological assessment to accurately quantify cognitive deficits and provide information about likely causes of the cognitive dysfunction.

Notably, there are few studies that have used specialised and specific neuropsychological assessment measures in patients with diabetic foot complications. The Marseglia et al. [43] MMSE study described above, utilised a small number of focussed neuropsychological assessment tasks, in addition to cognitive screening, in their predominantly male, diabetic foot cohort. This included the Trail Making Test A & B assessing processing speed and mental flexibility, the Rey Auditory Verbal Learning Test assessing verbal memory and Ravens Coloured Progressive Matrices assessing visual reasoning skills. The overall group means, and their deviation from expected premorbid or average age-matched norms, were not reported. However, age stratified data was provided and indicated that mental flexibility/set shifting, short-term verbal recall, processing speed and visual abstract reasoning were poorer in participants over 65 years of age. Logistic regression of disease factors indicated that HbA1c levels correlated with verbal memory difficulties in all patients, and that concurrent microvascular complications, and prior amputation was associated with verbal memory attenuation in patients over 65 years of age.

A further study by Kloos et al., attempted to determine if there was an association between foot ulcer relapse rate and cognitive impairment in 59 people with diabetes and previous foot ulcers [44]. The authors found no association between cognitive performance and re-ulceration at 1 year follow-up. However, a very limited number of neuropsychology tasks were employed in this study, assessing functioning only in the areas of vocabulary knowledge, perceptual logic and processing speed. There were no tasks assessing attention, memory or executive functioning. The follow-up period was also relatively short at 12 months, and no information was provided about re-ulceration in the three patients who died during the follow-up period.

The most comprehensive study to investigate neurocognitive functioning in diabetic foot patients using a broad assessment battery was undertaken by Natovich and colleagues in 2016 [46]. To date, this is the only published study that has used a wide-range multi-domain neuropsychological assessment battery to investigate neurocognitive functioning specifically in a diabetic foot ulcer cohort. This study investigated neurocognitive functioning in a group of 99 individuals with diabetic foot ulcers, along with a comparison group of 95 people with type 2 diabetes without foot ulcers. The study design incorporated the use of a computerised cognitive testing battery, NeuroTrax, with two more commonly used pencil and paper cognitive assessment tasks (Digit-symbol substitution task from the Wechsler Adult Intelligence Scale, WAIS; and a verbal fluency task).

The two late-middle aged study groups in Natovich et al. [46] were broadly matched on demographic and health related factors. This included gender ratio (predominantly male), smoking status and depressive symptoms. However, the non-foot ulcer group were slightly older, more highly educated, and had better diabetes control than their foot-ulcer counterparts, including significantly lower HbA1c scores, and lower hypertension, retinopathy, neuropathy, nephropathy and microvascular disease prevalence.

The neurocognitive test results from this study were age and education adjusted, in order to mitigate any impact of the mild cohort imbalances in these demographic factors [46]. The results on the NeuroTrax battery and additional pencil and paper tasks indicated significantly poorer cognitive functioning in participants with foot ulcers, compared to the non-foot ulcer group, across all activities assessing current cognitive functioning. This included scores in domains described as memory, attention and concentration, reaction time, executive functioning (with the description indicating predominantly a task of response inhibition), psychomotor speed, verbal fluency (phonemic and semantic), digit-symbol substitution, and global cognitive score (mean of domains, minus non-verbal intelligence). Post hoc adjustment for multiple comparisons was not reported in the study paper. However, when a Bonferroni correction is applied to the data, these group differences remain significant (i.e. $p < 0.005$). The only task on which a significant difference was not observed, was that estimating premorbid cognitive functioning (i.e. cognitive skills prior to any acquired neurocognitive impairment). It was further reported that global cognitive scores of the foot ulcer group differed significantly, from their estimated premorbid functioning, while the non-foot ulcer group did not. This appears to indicate generalised cognitive attenuation in the foot ulcer group.

A second important factor to consider from the data reported in the Natovich et al. [46], study is the magnitude of the differences between the foot ulcer group scores in each of the cognitive areas, relative to their estimated premorbid baseline. The results were normalised to a standard distribution (i.e. a mean score of 100–50th percentile, and standard deviation of 15–34 percentile ranks). The estimated premorbid cognition score for the foot ulcer group is reported as 96.78, which places at the 42nd percentile. None of the current cognitive functioning scores for the foot ulcer group were close to matching this. The current functioning score means ranged from as low as the 4th percentile (standard score of 72.77) for phonemic verbal fluency, to the 30th percentile (standard score of 91.76) for reaction time, with all but two results falling in the lowest quartile of functioning, for the age group. This contrasted with the non-foot ulcer group where the biggest percentile difference with premorbid cognition was 16 percentile ranks (standard score of 94.16 verses 100.19; 34th verses 50th percentile). With six out of the nine cognitive areas reported scoring within 5 percentile ranks of the premorbid estimate for this group. This indicates that attenuation in cognitive functioning in the foot ulcer group is at magnitudes of clinical significance for all cognitive areas, and likely to represent significant impairment in a number of individuals. The results also show the cognitive attenuation is generalised across areas and occurs relative to estimated premorbid abilities, age-matched normative data, and non-foot ulcer diabetic peers.

This study is a useful addition to the literature, as the first to examine neurocognitive functioning in a relatively comprehensive way, in a medium to large sample of individuals with diabetic foot ulcers. The researchers also attempted to match the sample, as closely as possible, with a non-foot ulcer diabetes comparison group. However, there are several limitations of the Natovich et al. study [46]. The first is the use of a less commonly used computerised measure of cognitive functioning, NeuroTrax. Although this measure has been reported on since 2003 the program appears to have been developed on a small normative sample, and its applicability outside studies of mild cognitive impairment and Parkinson's disease remains unclear [57, 58]. It is also unclear from the Natovich paper [46] exactly how NeuroTrax assesses functioning in each of the cognitive areas reported. For example, it is not clear what form the memory assessment takes (e.g. word list learning, narrative stories, paired associates), and this limits its comparability to other neuropsychological and diabetes research. It would have also been useful for the authors of this study to have provided information about the percentage individuals with neurocognitive dysfunction pronounced enough to meet the criteria for dementia. An additional limitation is the data in the study are taken from a single cross-sectional time point. The field would significantly benefit from research that takes a longitudinal approach to cognitive functioning in individuals with diabetic foot ulcers to determine if the development of cognitive attenuation precedes the development of foot ulcers, or vice-versa.

3.3 Theoretical framework of neurocognitive dysfunction in diabetic foot

The results from the Natovich et al. [46], study appear to support the earlier hypothesis proposed by Biessels and colleagues [3], of cognitive ageing and diabetes comorbidities acting as correlating or catalytic factors for diabetes related cognitive deterioration. The foot ulcer group in the Natovich et al. [46] study had a mean age of 58.04 years (SD 6.87). Research indicates that normal age related cognitive decline is demonstrated from as early as 45 years onwards, and most prominently occurs in the cognitive areas of visual spatial ability, processing speed, and fine motor skills [59]. Further, the foot-ulcer group had a considerably higher level of diabetes disease burden and comorbidity relative to the non-foot ulcer diabetes comparison group, with higher HbA1c scores, and significantly increased rates of retinopathy (51.5% vs. 9.5%), neuropathy (88.9% vs. 15.8%), nephropathy (33.3% vs. 3.2%) and micro-vascular disease (88.9% vs. 51.6%). The results of the cognitive screening study by Corbett et al. [45] also support the idea proposed by Biessels et al. [3], with cognitive attenuation seen above expectation for age in a late 50s cohort of diabetes foot ulcer patients, with high rates of comorbidity including hypertension, retinopathy and neuropathy. Thus, diabetic foot wounds could be argued to be an important risk variable for cognitive decline in middle-aged people with diabetes.

In **Figure 1**, a graphical representation has been provided to visually illustrate the impact of diabetes, across the lifespan, for Type 1 diabetes, Type 2 diabetes, and people with diabetic foot complications, relative to normal functioning. The graph provides a representation of generalised cognitive proficiency (summed across cognitive domains) and illustrates what is known about neurocognitive functioning

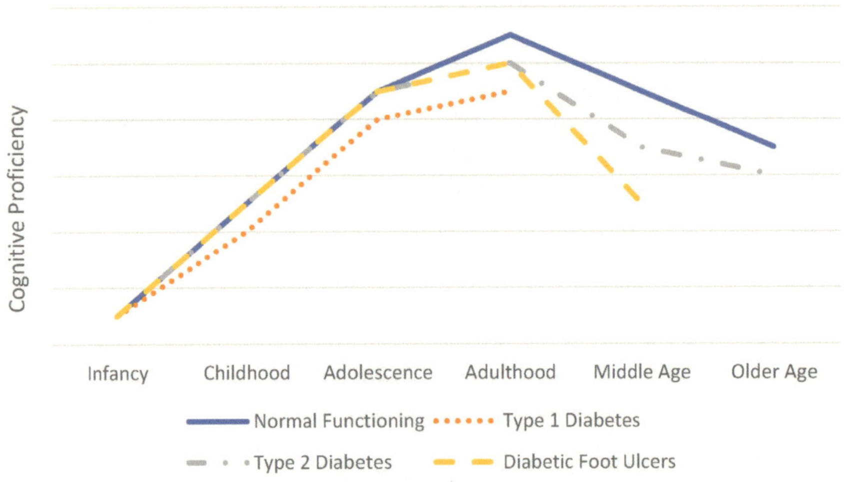

Figure 1.
Neurocognitive functioning across the lifespan.

in each of the groups, based on the currently available literature. Further research is needed to definitively characterise the magnitude of neurocognitive decline in individuals with diabetic foot ulcers, and also to determine if there are any differences in the rates and types of decline in Type 1 versus Type 2 suffers. Additional research would also be beneficial into neurocognitive functioning in Type 1 cohorts into middle and older age, as currently there are few studies that include Type 1 patients in these age groups.

3.4 Self-management

The available neurocognitive functioning results in diabetic foot ulcer samples raise a number of concerns about the capacity of this group to effectively implement self-management practices. Self-management requires the ability to adequately understand, process and recall recommendations, as well as to consistently implement these effectively in daily life. Given the rates of pronounced cognitive decrement that appear to be present in a number of diabetic people with foot wounds, it could be expected that a sizable proportion of this cohort may lack the capacity to do this. Interestingly, in 2017 a second study was published by the Natovich lead study group, that compared adherence to self-care in two diabetes samples, those with and without foot ulcers [60]. Although not specifically stated by the authors, this study appears to have utilised the same cohort of participants and controls to their neurocognitive study, described above [46], as the reported sample numbers and demographic details of participants are the same. This study employed the Summary of Diabetes Self-Care Activity self-report scale as well as two objective measures of diabetes control and adherence (BMI and HbA1C levels). The results indicated that individuals with foot ulcers were more adherent to blood tests, but less adherent to physical activity recommendations and had poor glycaemic control (HbA1c). The authors speculated that this may be due to difficulty in linking problematic glycaemic test results to changes in actual behaviour, as a result of cognitive impairment. They also suggested that the reduced physical activity in the foot-ulcer group may make glycaemic levels more difficult to control. The cognitive screening study by Corbett and colleagues [45] indicated that individuals with foot ulcers and lower cognitive functioning had reduced understanding of how foot wounds occur, relative to cognitively higher functioning participants. It would be interesting for this to be investigated further to determine if these individuals are at higher likelihood of experiencing poorer wound healing and re-ulceration in the future.

4. Conclusion

The available evidence indicates that neurocognitive dysfunction in individuals with diabetic foot ulcers is more pronounced than expected, for both their age and diabetes status. Thus, diabetic foot complications appear to be associated with cognitive impairment. The mechanistic causes of this dysfunction is likely to be related to the overall poorer diabetes control in this group, including higher HbA1c scores, and higher rates of hypertension, retinopathy, neuropathy, nephropathy and microvascular disease, relative to diabetes peers without foot ulcers. Many of these complications have been found to contribute to an increase in the prevalence of vascular dementia and Alzheimer's disease in people with diabetes. Thus, cognitive impairment in this group may represent disease burden caused by a combination of glycaemic and vascular factors, leading to accelerated neuronal death. Cognitive impairment may contribute to a 'vicious cycle' reducing the capacity of people to effectively self-manage their diabetes and foot health, which in turn results in poorer diabetes control and an increase in complications, leading to further attenuation in cognitive functioning.

More research is needed to provide further information about the cognitive profile of individuals with diabetic foot ulcers, using a large battery of commonly utilised clinical neuropsychology assessment measures. The four existing studies have provided some useful initial information. However, additional work clearly outlining the specific domains of cognitive impairment, and the magnitude of this impairment, using commonly utilised neuropsychological tests, is required. Longitudinal research to determine whether cognitive decline increases over time in this group would be useful. Combining cognitive functioning measures with neuroimaging in the same cohort would also help to determine if cognitive impairment is associated with observable neurological abnormalities. Including psychological factors, such as the high frequency mental health conditions of depression and anxiety, as well as diabetes distress ratings, would provide information about whether psychological factors also impact on cognitive functioning, and potentially treatment adherence in this group.

Routine cognitive screening is likely to be beneficial in individuals with diabetic foot ulcers, as the available evidence indicates a high proportion will have cognitive dysfunction. Where available, individuals showing moderate to significant difficulties on screening measures should be referred for clinical neuropsychological assessment, to quantify the magnitude and specific nature of their cognitive difficulties. Neuropsychologists can also provide an individualised plan for cognitive remediation and management strategies to assist with cognitive difficulties in daily life. This may assist in improving effective self-management compliance and improve over outcomes in his group.

Conflict of interest

The authors declare no conflict of interest.

Author details

Caroline A. Fisher[1,2]

1 Allied Health – Psychology, Royal Melbourne Hospital, Melbourne, Victoria, Australia

2 The Melbourne Clinic, Melbourne, Victoria, Australia

*Address all correspondence to: caroline.fisher2@mh.org.au

References

[1] Katsarou A, Gudbjörnsdottir S, Rawshani A, Dabelea D, Bonifacio E, Anderson BJ, et al. Type 1 diabetes mellitus. Nature Reviews. Disease Primers. 2017;**3**:1-18

[2] Atkinson M, Eisenbarth G, Michels A. Type 1 diabetes. Lancet. 2014;**383**(9911):69-82

[3] Biessels GJ, Deary IJ, Ryan CM. Cognition and diabetes: A lifespan perspective. Lancet Neurology. 2008;**7**(2):184-190

[4] Zheng Y, Ley SH, Hu FB. Global aetiology and epidemiology of type 2 diabetes mellitus and its complications. Nature Reviews Endocrinology. 2018;**14**:88-98

[5] Cnop M, Welsh N, Jonas J-C, Jorns A, Lenzen S, Eizirik DL. Mechanisms of pancreatic β-cell death in Type 1 and Type 2 diabetes: Many differences, few similarities. Diabetes. 2005;**54**:S97-S107

[6] Dabelea D, Mayer-Davis E, Saydah S, Imperatore G, Linder B, Divers J, et al. Prevalence of Type 1 and Type 2 diabetes among children and adolescents from 2001 to 2009 Dana. JAMA: The Journal of the American Medical Association. 2014;**311**(17):1778-1786

[7] NCD Risk Factor Collaboration. Worldwide trends in diabetes since 1980: A pooled analysis of 751 population-based studies with 4.4 million participants. Lancet. 2016;**387**(10027):1513-1530

[8] Jeffcoate WJ, Harding KG. Diabetic foot ulcers. Lancet. 2003;**361**(May 3): 1545-1551

[9] Boulton AJ, Vileikyte L, Ragnarson-Tennvall G, Apelqvist J. The global burden of diabetic foot disease. Lancet. 2005;**366**(9498):1719-1724

[10] Armstrong DG, Boulton AJM, Bus SA. Diabetic foot ulcers and their recurrence. The New England Journal of Medicine. 2017;**376**(24):2367-2375

[11] Prompers L, Schaper N, Apelqvist J, Edmonds MJ, Ude E, Mauricio D, et al. Prediction of outcome in individuals with diabetic foot ulcers: Focus on the differences between individuals with and without peripheral arterial disease: The EURODIALE Study. Diabetologia. 2008;**51**:747-755

[12] Zhang P, Lu J, Jing Y, Tang S, Zhu D, Bi Y. Global epidemiology of diabetic foot ulceration: A systematic review and meta-analysis. Annals of Medicine. 2017;**49**(2):106-116

[13] Lepäntalo M, Apelqvist J, Setacci C, Ricco J, De Donato G, Becker F, et al. Chapter V: Diabetic foot. European Journal of Vascular and Endovascular Surgery. 2011;**42**(Dec 1):S60-S74

[14] Walsh J, Hoffstad O, Sullivan M, Margolis DJ. Association of diabetic foot ulcer and death in a population-based cohort from the United Kingdom. Diabetic Medicine. 2016;**33**:1493-1498

[15] Boyko E, Ahroni J, Smith D, Davignon D. Increased mortality associated with diabetic foot ulcer. Diabetic Medicine. 1996;**13**:967-972

[16] Jeyaraman K, Berhane T, Hamilton M, Chandra AP, Falhammar H. Mortality in patients with diabetic foot ulcer: A retrospective study of 513 cases from a single Centre in the Northern Territory of Australia. BMC Endocrine Disorders. 2019;**19**(1):1-7

[17] Goodridge D, Trepman E, Embil JM. Health-related quality of life in diabetic patients with foot ulcers: Literature review. Journal of Wound, Ostomy, and Continence Nursing. 2005;**32**(6):368-377

[18] Meusel LC, Kansal N, Tchistiakova E, Yuen W. A systematic review of type 2 diabetes mellitus and hypertension in imaging studies of cognitive aging: Time to establish new norms. Frontiers in Aging Neuroscience. 2014;**6**(July):1-17

[19] Schmidt R, Launer L, Nilsson L-G, Pajak A, Sans S, Berger K, et al. Magnetic resonance imaging of the brain in diabetes. 2004;**53**:687-692

[20] Hankey GJ, Anderson NE, Ting RD, Veillard AS, Romo M, Wosik M, et al. Rates and predictors of risk of stroke and its subtypes in diabetes: A prospective observational study. Journal of Neurology, Neurosurgery, and Psychiatry. 2013;**84**(3):281-287

[21] Geijselaers SLC. Cognitive Dysfunction: At the Crossroads of Glucose Metabolism and Vascular Function. Maastricht: Maastricht University; 2016

[22] Van Harten B, De Leeuw FE, Weinstein HC, Scheltens P, Biessels GJ. Brain imaging in patients with diabetes: A systematic review. Diabetes Care. 2006;**29**(11):2539-2548

[23] Biessels GJ, Reijmer YD. Brain changes underlying cognitive dysfunction in diabetes: What can we learn from MRI? Diabetes. 2014;**63**(7):2244-2252

[24] Macpherson H, Formica M, Harris E, Daly RM. Brain functional alterations in Type 2 diabetes—A systematic review of fMRI studies. Frontiers in Neuroendocrinology. 2017;**47**(June 2017):34-46

[25] Funnell MM, Brown TL, Childs BP, Haas LB, Hosey GM, Jensen B, et al. National standards for diabetes self-management education. Diabetes Care. 2008;**31**:S97-S104

[26] Kisokanth G, Prathapan S, Indrakumar J, Joseph J. Factors influencing self-management of diabetes mellitus: A review article. Journal of Diabetology. 2013;**3**(1):1-7

[27] Funnell MM, Anderson RM. Empowerment and self-management of diabetes. Clinical Diabetes. 2004;**22**(3):123-127

[28] Haas L, Maryniuk M, Beck J, Cox CE, Duker P, Edwards L, et al. National standards for diabetes self-management education and support. Diabetes Care. 2012;**35**:2393-2401

[29] Lin A, Northam EA, Rankins D, Werther GA, Cameron FJ. Neuropsychological profiles of young people with type 1 diabetes 12 yr after disease onset. Pediatric Diabetes. 2010;**11**(4):235-243

[30] Spauwen PJJ, Köhler S, Verhey FRJ, Stehouwer CDA, Van Boxtel MPJ. Effects of type 2 diabetes on 12-year cognitive change: Results from the Maastricht Aging Study. Diabetes Care. 2013;**36**(6):1554-1561

[31] Mori Y, Futamura A, Murakami H, Kohashi K, Hirano T, Kawamura M. Increased detection of mild cognitive impairment with type 2 diabetes mellitus using the Japanese version of the Montreal Cognitive Assessment: A pilot study. Neurology and Clinical Neuroscience. 2015;**3**(3):89-93

[32] Ogurel T, Oȷurel R, Özer M, Türkel Y, Daȷ E, Örnek K. Mini-mental state exam versus Montreal Cognitive Assessment in patients with diabetic retinopathy. Nigerian Journal of Clinical Practice. 2015;**18**(6):786-789

[33] Ojo O, Brooke J. Evaluating the association between diabetes, cognitive decline and dementia. International Journal of Environmental Research and Public Health. 2015;**12**:8281-8294

[34] Chatterjee S, Peters SAE, Woodward M, Arango SM, Batty GD,

Beckett N, et al. Type 2 diabetes as a risk factor for dementia in women compared with men: A pooled analysis of 2.3 million people comprising more than 100,000 cases of dementia. Diabetes Care. 2016;**39**(2):300-307

[35] Ahtiluoto S, Polvikoski T, Peltonen M, Solomon A, Tuomilehto J, Winblad B, et al. Diabetes, Alzheimer disease, and vascular dementia. Neurology. 2010;**75**(13):1195-1202

[36] American Psychiatric Association. Diagnostic and Statistical Manual of Mental Disorders (DSM-5®). USA: American Psychiatric Pub; 2013

[37] McCrimmon RJ, Ryan CM, Frier BM. Diabetes and cognitive dysfunction. Lancet. 2012;**379**(9833):2291-2299

[38] Brands AM, Biessels GJ, De Haan EH, Kappelle LJ, Kessels RP. The effects of type 1 diabetes on cognitive performance. Diabetes Care. 2005;**28**(2005):726-733

[39] Ruis C, Biessels GJ, Gorter KJ, Van Den Donk M, Kappelle LJ, Rutten GEHM. Cognition in the early stage of type 2 diabetes. Diabetes Care. 2009;**32**(7):1261-1265

[40] Palta P, Schneider ALC, Biessels GJ, Touradji P, Hill-Briggs F. Magnitude of cognitive dysfunction in adults with type 2 diabetes: A meta-analysis of six cognitive domains and the most frequently reported neuropsychological tests within domains. Journal of the International Neuropsychological Society. 2014;**20**(3):278-291

[41] Chen Y, Liu Z, Wang A, Zhang J, Zhang S, Qi D, et al. Dysfunctional organization of default mode network before memory impairments in type 2 diabetes. Psychoneuroendocrinology. 2016;**74**(2016):141-148

[42] Cui Y, Jiao Y, Chen YC, Wang K, Gao B, Wen S, et al. Altered spontaneous brain activity in type 2 diabetes: A resting-state functional MRI study. Diabetes. 2014;**63**(2):749-760

[43] Marseglia A, Xu W, Rizzuto D, Ferrari C, Whisstock C, Brocco E, et al. Cognitive functioning among patients with diabetic foot. Journal of Diabetes and its Complications. 2014;**28**(6):863-868

[44] Kloos C, Hagen F, Lindloh C, Braun A, Leppert K, Muller N, et al. Recurrent foot ulcers in patients with diabetes and neuropathy. Diabetes Care. 2009;**32**(5):894-896

[45] Corbett C, Jolley J, Barson E, Wraight P, Perrin B, Fisher C. Cognition and understanding of neuropathy of inpatients admitted to a specialized tertiary diabetic foot unit with diabetes-related foot ulcers. The International Journal of Lower Extremity Wounds. 2019;**18**(3):294-300

[46] Natovich R, Kushnir T, Harman-Boehm I, Margalit D, Siev-Ner I, Tsalichin D, et al. Cognitive dysfunction: Part and parcel of the diabetic foot. Diabetes Care. 2016;**39**(7):1202-1207

[47] Folstein M, Folstein S, McHugh P. Mini-mental state: A practical method of grading the cognitive state of patients for the clinician. Journal of Psychiatric Research. 1975;**12**:189-198

[48] Kivipelto M, Helkala EL, Hänninen T, Laakso MP, Hallikainen M, Alhainen K, et al. Midlife vascular risk factors and late-life mild cognitive impairment: A population-based study. Neurology. 2001;**56**(12):1683-1689

[49] Trzepacz PT, Hochstetler H, Wang S, Walker B, Saykin AJ. Relationship between the Montreal cognitive assessment and mini-mental state examination for assessment of mild cognitive impairment in older adults. BMC Geriatrics. 2015;**15**(1):1-9

[50] Nasreddine ZS, Phillips NA, Bédirian V, Charbonneau S, Whitehead V, Collin I, et al. The Montreal Cognitive Assessment, MoCA: A brief screening tool for mild cognitive impairment. Journal of the American Geriatrics Society. 2005;**53**(2):695-699

[51] Carson N, Leach L, Murphy KJ. A re-examination of Montreal Cognitive Assessment (MoCA) cutoff scores. International Journal of Geriatric Psychiatry. 2018;**33**(2):379-388

[52] Smith T, Gildeh N, Holmes C. Validity and utility in a memory clinic setting. Revue. 2007;**52**(5):329-332

[53] Costa AS, Reich A, Fimm B, Ketteler ST, Schulz JB, Reetz K. Evidence of the sensitivity of the MoCA alternate forms in monitoring cognitive change in early Alzheimer's disease. Dementia and Geriatric Cognitive Disorders. 2014;**37**(1-2):95-103

[54] Özcan T, Demir EY. Investigation the cognitive impairment in diabetes mellitus type 2 with moca test. African Journal of Psychiatry (South Africa). 2014;**17**(6):13-15

[55] Alagiakrishnan K, Zhao N, Mereu L, Senior P, Senthilselvan A. Montreal cognitive assessment is superior to standardized mini-mental status exam in detecting mild cognitive impairment in the middle-aged and elderly patients with type 2 diabetes mellitus. BioMed Research International. 2013;**2013**:1-5

[56] Karan SN. Assessment of the cognitive status in diabetes mellitus. Journal of Clinical and Diagnostic Research. 2012;**6**(10):1658-1662

[57] Dwolatzky T, Whitehead V, Doniger GM, Simon ES, Schweiger A, Jaffe D, et al. Validity of a novel computerized cognitive battery for mild cognitive impairment. BMC Geriatrics. 1 Dec 2003;**3**(1):4

[58] Schweiger A, Doniger GM, Dwolatzky T, Jaffe D, Simon E. Reliability of a novel computerized neuropsychological battery for mild cognitive impairment. Acta Neuropsychologica. 2003;**1**:407-413

[59] Hoogendam YY, Hofman A, Van Der Geest JN, Van Der Lugt A, Ikram MA. Patterns of cognitive function in aging: The Rotterdam Study. European Journal of Epidemiology. 2014;**29**(2):133-140

[60] Natovich R, Harman-boehm I, Margalit D, Cukierman T. Adherence to self-care among individuals with diabetes with and without diabetic foot complications: Objective and self-report measures. Diabetes Management. 2017;7:234-239